Wholesome Plant-Centric Cuisine

Flavorful Recipes and Practical Tips

Len Glover

<u>Copyrights</u>

Table of contents

Introduction

The Plant-Centric Eating

It The Plant-Centric Eating (PCE) lifestyle has gained considerable attention in recent years, advocating for a diet primarily composed of minimally processed plant foods. This dietary approach emphasizes the consumption of fruits, vegetables, whole grains, legumes, nuts, and seeds while avoiding or minimizing animal products and processed foods. This lifestyle not only addresses health concerns but also promotes environmental sustainability and animal welfare.

One of the key benefits of the PCE lifestyle is its positive impact on health. Research suggests that such a diet can lower the risk of chronic diseases like heart disease, diabetes, and certain types of cancer. The abundance of vitamins, minerals, and antioxidants found in plant foods contributes to improved overall well-being and reduced inflammation. Moreover, the high fiber content aids digestion and supports weight management.

Environmental considerations also play a significant role in adopting a PCE lifestyle. Plant-based diets have a lower carbon footprint compared to diets centered around animal agriculture. Animal farming requires substantial resources, including land, water, and energy. By choosing plant-based options, individuals can contribute to reducing their ecological footprint and mitigating the effects of climate change.

Ethical concerns surrounding animal welfare further contribute to the appeal of the PCE lifestyle. Advocates of this lifestyle argue that minimizing animal product consumption aligns with the principles of compassion and reduces the demand for industries that often raise animals in confined and unnatural conditions.

Transitioning to a PCE lifestyle requires careful planning and consideration to ensure adequate nutrient intake. While plant-based diets offer numerous benefits, individuals need to pay attention to sources of essential nutrients like protein, iron, vitamin B12, calcium, and omega-3 fatty acids. A well-balanced approach involves consuming a variety of plant foods and, if necessary, considering fortified foods or supplements.

Plant-Centric Eating offers a holistic approach to health, sustainability, and ethics. By focusing on consuming minimally processed plant foods and reducing the consumption of animal products, individuals can potentially enhance their well-being, reduce their environmental impact, and contribute to the ethical treatment of animals. However, it's crucial to approach this lifestyle with knowledge and proper planning to ensure a balanced and nutritious diet.

<u>Benefits of Minimal Ingredients</u>

Cooking with minimal ingredients is not only a practical approach but also a creative and fulfilling way to prepare meals. Embracing simplicity in the kitchen can offer a range of advantages that go beyond just saving time and effort. Here are some key benefits of cooking with minimal ingredients:

1. Time-Saving: One of the most obvious benefits of cooking with minimal ingredients is the time it saves. With fewer components to prepare and combine, the cooking process becomes quicker and more efficient. This is especially helpful on busy days when you need to put together a meal without spending hours in the kitchen.

2. Cost-Effective: Cooking with fewer ingredients often translates to spending less money on groceries. By focusing on a handful of staple items, you can reduce food waste and make the most of what you have. This can lead to significant savings over time.

3. Enhanced Flavors: When you work with a limited number of ingredients, you're more likely to pay attention to their quality and how they interact with each other. This can result in dishes with well-balanced and heightened flavors, where each ingredient plays a vital role.

4. Creativity and Innovation: Minimalist cooking encourages creativity in the kitchen. With limited ingredients, you'll find yourself experimenting and thinking outside the box to create unique and delicious dishes. This can help you develop your culinary skills and discover new flavor combinations.

5. Less Clutter: Keeping your pantry and refrigerator stocked with fewer items not only reduces clutter but also makes it easier to stay organized. You'll be able to see what you have on hand more clearly, preventing duplicate purchases and reducing food waste.

6. Healthier Choices: Minimal ingredient cooking often leads to healthier choices. You're more likely to use fresh, whole foods and avoid highly processed options that are loaded with additives and preservatives. This can contribute to a more balanced and nutritious diet.

7. Reduced Food Waste: With a focus on using what you have, you'll be less likely to let ingredients go to waste. This is an eco-friendly approach that helps minimize your impact on the environment.

8. Stress Reduction: Simplifying your cooking process by using minimal ingredients can reduce stress in the kitchen. It eliminates the need to follow complex recipes and juggle numerous components, making cooking a more enjoyable and relaxing experience.

9. Portion Control: Cooking with minimal ingredients can naturally lead to portion control. You'll prepare just the right amount of food without feeling overwhelmed by leftovers that might go uneaten.

10. Quick Meal Solutions: Minimal ingredient cooking is ideal for those times when you need to whip up a meal in a hurry. By relying on a few key ingredients, you can create satisfying and nutritious dishes without spending too much time on preparation.

Cooking with minimal ingredients offers a host of benefits, from saving time and money to encouraging creativity and healthier eating habits. Embracing simplicity in the kitchen can lead to delicious meals that are both satisfying and rewarding to prepare.

Flavorful Meals without Salt

1. Herbs and Spices: Use a variety of fresh and dried herbs, spices, and seasonings to add depth and complexity to your dishes. Examples include garlic, ginger, cumin, paprika, turmeric, and oregano.

2. Citrus: Enhance flavors with citrus fruits like lemon, lime, and orange. Their natural acidity can brighten up your dishes and provide a tangy kick.

3. Vinegar: Experiment with different types of vinegar, such as balsamic, apple cider, and rice vinegar, to bring a zesty flavor to your meals.

4. Natural Sweeteners: Opt for natural sweeteners like dates, maple syrup, honey, or mashed ripe bananas to add sweetness without refined sugar.

5. Roasting and Grilling: Roasting or grilling vegetables and proteins can bring out natural flavors and create caramelization without the need for oil.

6. Broths and Stocks: Use homemade or low-sodium vegetable or mushroom broth as a flavorful base for soups, stews, and sauces.

7. Nuts and Seeds: Incorporate crushed nuts and seeds like almonds, walnuts, and sunflower seeds for a satisfying crunch and a boost of flavor.

8. Creamy Textures: Create creamy textures by using ingredients like avocado, unsweetened coconut milk, or blended silken tofu.

9. Umami-rich Foods: Include umami-packed ingredients like mushrooms, tomatoes, miso paste, nutritional yeast, and soy sauce (in moderation) to enhance savory flavors.

10. Fresh Herbs: Garnish your dishes with fresh herbs like basil, cilantro, parsley, or mint to add a burst of freshness and aroma.

11. Texture Contrast: Play with different textures by incorporating crisp vegetables, tender grains, and chewy legumes to create a satisfying eating experience.

12. Marination: Allow your proteins or vegetables to marinate in flavorful mixtures, such as a combination of citrus juice, herbs, and spices, before cooking.

13. Cooking Techniques: Explore techniques like sautéing, steaming, and braising to retain and amplify natural flavors.

Breakfast Delights

The sun's gentle rays cast a warm glow as a new day awakens, and with it comes the promise of a delightful breakfast that fuels both body and soul. A symphony of scents drifts from the kitchen, mingling with the anticipation that lingers in the air.

As the aroma of freshly brewed coffee dances in the air, it's a wake-up call to the senses, a signal that the day has officially begun. The rich, earthy notes of the coffee beans tempt even the most reluctant risers out of their slumber, promising a jolt of energy to kickstart the morning.

Meanwhile, the sizzle of eggs hitting the pan forms a savory symphony, accompanied by the crisp crunch of bacon and the gentle hiss of buttery toast browning to perfection. These familiar sounds are the soundtrack of comfort, reassuring us that the morning routine is unfolding just as it should.

For those with a sweet tooth, breakfast offers an array of delights. Fluffy pancakes, adorned with a drizzle of golden maple syrup, provide a decadent treat that brings back memories of lazy weekend mornings. The vibrant hues of fresh berries burst forth from bowls of yogurt, adding a burst of color and a touch of healthful sweetness.

In the world of breakfast, cultures collide, offering a diverse array of options that cater to every palate. A traditional Japanese breakfast might feature miso soup, rice, grilled fish, and pickled vegetables. Meanwhile, a Mexican breakfast might embrace the hearty flavors of huevos rancheros, while India's parathas with spicy chutneys awaken the taste buds.

Breakfast is not only about sustenance; it's a ritual of connection. Families gather around the table, sharing stories and laughter as they savor the first meal of the day together. Friends catch up over steaming cups of tea, and colleagues discuss the day ahead while nibbling on flaky pastries.

Yet, breakfast delights extend beyond the boundaries of the familiar. Cafés and bistros entice with artisanal creations, like avocado toast topped with poached eggs or artisanal pastries filled with unexpected flavors. With each bite, a journey of exploration begins, as old favorites are revisited and discoveries are made.

In a world that moves at a relentless pace, breakfast remains a timeless indulgence, a chance to pause and embrace the simple pleasures of life. Whether it's a leisurely feast that stretches into late morning or a quick bite on the go, breakfast delights offer a daily reminder that the best things in life often begin with a humble meal.

Here are some common breakfast delights:

1. Scrambled eggs
2. Bacon or sausage
3. Pancakes or waffles
4. Toast with butter and jam
5. Cereal with milk
6. Omelette with various fillings
7. Fresh fruit (e.g., berries, bananas)
8. Yogurt with granola
9. Croissants or pastries
10. Breakfast burritos
11. Smoothies
12. Avocado toast
13. Hash browns
14. Bagels with cream cheese
15. Breakfast sandwiches

<u>Quick Oatmeal with Fresh Berries</u>

When it comes to a nourishing and delightful breakfast, few dishes can compare to a steaming bowl of quick oatmeal topped with an assortment of fresh berries. This simple yet satisfying meal is not only a treat for the taste buds but also a source of essential nutrients that kickstart your day on the right note.

Preparing quick oatmeal with fresh berries is a breeze, making it a perfect option for those rushed mornings. To begin, gather your ingredients: quick-cooking oats, water or milk (dairy or plant-based), a pinch of salt, a touch of sweetener (like honey or maple syrup), and a variety of fresh berries such as strawberries, blueberries, raspberries, or blackberries.

The cooking process is as effortless as it gets. Start by heating the water or milk in a saucepan until it reaches a gentle boil. Add the quick-cooking oats and a pinch of salt, stirring occasionally to prevent sticking. Within minutes, the oats will soften and thicken, creating a creamy base for your breakfast.

Now, for the delightful twist: the fresh berries. As the oatmeal simmers, wash and prepare a handful of your chosen berries. Their vibrant colors and natural sweetness will infuse your meal with a burst of flavor and a pop of antioxidants. Once the oats are cooked to your desired consistency, transfer them to a serving bowl.

With your bowl of warm oatmeal ready, it's time to adorn it with luscious berries. Gently scatter the fresh berries over the oatmeal, allowing their juices to meld with the creamy oats. Drizzle a touch of your preferred sweetener to enhance the overall taste. The contrasting textures of the velvety oatmeal and the juicy berries create a delightful symphony of flavors in every spoonful.

Aside from its delectable taste, this quick oatmeal with fresh berries is a nutritional powerhouse. Oats are rich in dietary fiber, which aids digestion and keeps you feeling full for longer. Berries, on the other hand, are loaded with vitamins, minerals, and antioxidants that promote overall health and well-being. This breakfast combination provides a balanced mix of carbohydrates, protein, and healthy fats, giving you sustained energy to tackle your day.

The marriage of quick oatmeal and fresh berries is a harmonious blend of convenience and nutrition. With minimal effort, you can prepare a heartwarming bowl of oatmeal that not only satisfies your taste buds but also nourishes your body. So, on those mornings when time is of the essence, remember this delightful recipe and relish the goodness it brings to your breakfast table.

<u>Itemized Process for Quick Oatmeal with Fresh Berries</u>

1. Gather Ingredients:

- Quick oats

- Water or milk (your choice)

- Fresh berries (e.g., strawberries, blueberries, raspberries)

- Sweetener (optional)

- Nuts or seeds (optional)

- Cinnamon or other spices (optional)

2. Measure Oats and Liquid:

- Measure the desired amount of quick oats. Usually, 1/2 to 1 cup is a common serving size.

- Measure an equal amount of water or milk. The exact amount depends on your preferred oatmeal consistency.

3. Combine Oats and Liquid:

- In a microwave-safe bowl, mix the quick oats and liquid.

4. Cook in Microwave:

- Place the bowl in the microwave and cook on high for 1-2 minutes. Cooking time may vary based on microwave wattage and desired oatmeal thickness.

5. Stir and Add Sweetener:

- Carefully remove the bowl from the microwave (it will be hot) and give the oatmeal a good stir.

- If desired, add a sweetener like honey, maple syrup, or sugar. Adjust the amount to taste.

6. Add Fresh Berries:

- Wash and prepare the fresh berries. You can leave them whole or slice them, depending on your preference.

7. Top with Berries and Optional Ingredients:

- Add the fresh berries on top of the oatmeal. You can also add nuts, seeds, a sprinkle of cinnamon, or other spices for extra flavor and texture.

8. Serve and Enjoy:

- Your quick oatmeal with fresh berries is ready to enjoy! Be sure to let it cool slightly before eating.

<u>Quick Oatmeal with Fresh Berries Problems and solutions</u>

Problem: Soggy Texture - Quick oatmeal can become too mushy or have a soggy texture when prepared with fresh berries.

Solution: Add the fresh berries after cooking the oatmeal. This prevents them from releasing excess moisture and maintains a better texture.

<u>Problem: Tartness of Berries</u> - Some fresh berries can be tart, affecting the overall taste of the oatmeal.

Solution: Sweeten the oatmeal with honey, maple syrup, or a sprinkle of brown sugar to balance out the tartness of the berries.

<u>Problem: Berries Discoloration</u> - Fresh berries may release their juices and cause discoloration in the oatmeal.

Solution: Gently fold in the berries towards the end of cooking to minimize juice release. Alternatively, you can layer the berries on top after serving.

<u>Problem: Berry Selection</u> - Choosing the right berries is crucial, as some varieties might not pair well with oatmeal.

Solution: Opt for berries like strawberries, blueberries, or raspberries, which are commonly used in oatmeal due to their flavor and texture.

<u>Problem: Nutritional Balance - Quick oatmeal with fresh berries might lack protein and healthy fats.</u>

Solution: Enhance the nutritional profile by adding ingredients like chopped nuts, chia seeds, or a dollop of yogurt to provide additional protein and healthy fats.

Problem: Texture and Crunch - Quick oatmeal can sometimes lack texture and crunch.

Solution: Top the oatmeal with granola, toasted coconut flakes, or sliced almonds to add a pleasant crunch to each bite.

Problem: Overcooking Berries - Berries can easily overcook and lose their shape and flavor.

Solution: Use a gentle heat and cook the berries for a shorter time, or even consider making a quick berry compote separately and adding it to the oatmeal just before serving.

<u>Problem: Temperature</u> - If the berries are too cold, they can cool down the oatmeal quickly.

Solution: Allow the berries to come to room temperature before adding them to the oatmeal or warm them slightly in the microwave if needed.

<u>Problem: Seasonal Availability</u> - Fresh berries might not be readily available year-round.

Solution: Consider using frozen berries when fresh ones are out of season. Thaw them slightly before adding to the oatmeal.

Banana Walnut Muffins: A Delightful Blend of Flavors

Banana walnut muffins are a delightful treat that combines the sweetness of ripe bananas with the rich nuttiness of walnuts. These muffins are not only a popular choice for breakfast but also make for a wonderful snack throughout the day. The fusion of flavors and textures creates a harmonious experience that appeals to a wide range of palates.

At the heart of these muffins lies the star ingredient: ripe bananas. Their natural sweetness not only imparts a luscious taste but also contributes to the muffins' moist and tender crumb. The bananas also serve as a healthier alternative to excess sugar, making these muffins a guilt-free option for those watching their sugar intake.

Adding walnuts to the mix introduces a delightful crunch and earthy flavor that compliments the banana's sweetness. Walnuts are known for their numerous health benefits, including being a good source of omega-3 fatty acids and antioxidants. Their inclusion in these muffins not only enhances the taste but also adds a nutritious element.

The process of creating banana walnut muffins is a simple yet rewarding endeavor. A basic muffin batter is prepared by combining flour, baking powder, and a touch of salt. The mashed bananas are then folded into the batter, imparting their characteristic aroma and flavor. Chopped walnuts are added for the desired crunch and depth of taste. The batter is carefully scooped into muffin cups and baked until golden brown and fragrant.

The aroma that fills the kitchen as these muffins bake is truly inviting. The gentle scent of bananas and the toasty aroma of walnuts create an ambiance that awakens the senses. Once out of the oven, the muffins are allowed to cool slightly before being enjoyed.

These muffins offer versatility as well. They can be enjoyed as is, or you can elevate them by spreading a dollop of creamy butter or a drizzle of honey on top. They can be paired with a warm cup of coffee or tea, making them an ideal choice for a leisurely breakfast or a cozy afternoon break.

Banana walnut muffins are a harmonious fusion of flavors and textures that make for a delightful treat. The sweetness of ripe bananas and the nuttiness of walnuts come together to create a muffin that is not only tasty but also nutritious. Whether enjoyed as a breakfast option or a midday snack, these muffins are sure to leave a lasting impression on your taste buds.

Banana Walnut Muffin Recipe

Certainly! Here's an itemized process for preparing Banana Walnut Muffins:

1. Gather Ingredients:

- Ripe bananas (3)

- All-purpose flour (2 cups)

- Baking powder (1 tsp)

- Baking soda (1/2 tsp)

- Salt (1/4 tsp)

- Unsalted butter (1/2 cup, melted)

- Granulated sugar (3/4 cup)

- Eggs (2)

- Vanilla extract (1 tsp)

- Chopped walnuts (1/2 cup)

2. Preheat Oven:

Preheat your oven to 350°F (175°C). Prepare muffin tins by greasing or lining them with paper liners.

3. Mash Bananas:

In a bowl, mash the ripe bananas using a fork until smooth. Set aside.

4. Mix Dry Ingredients:

In a separate large bowl, whisk together the all-purpose flour, baking powder, baking soda, and salt.

5. Combine Wet Ingredients:

In another bowl, whisk together the melted butter and granulated sugar until well combined. Add the eggs one at a time, mixing well after each addition. Stir in the vanilla extract and mashed bananas.

6. Combine Wet and Dry Mixtures:

Pour the wet mixture into the dry mixture and gently fold until just combined. Do not overmix.

7. Add Chopped Walnuts:

Gently fold the chopped walnuts into the batter.

8. Fill Muffin Cups:

Using a spoon or an ice cream scoop, divide the batter evenly among the prepared muffin cups, filling each about 2/3 full.

9. Bake:

Place the muffin tin in the preheated oven and bake for about 18-20 minutes, or until a toothpick inserted into the center of a muffin comes out clean.

10. Cool and Enjoy:

Once baked, remove the muffins from the oven and allow them to cool in the tin for a few minutes before transferring them to a wire rack to cool completely. Enjoy your delightful Banana Walnut Muffins!

Every cooking time and temperature may vary, so keep an eye on your muffins as they bake. Enjoy your homemade treats!

<u>Banana Walnut Muffins Problems And Solutions</u>

By being mindful of these potential problems and applying the suggested solutions, you'll be better equipped to create a batch of delicious and perfectly baked Banana Walnut Muffins!

Here are some common problems that can arise while preparing Banana Walnut Muffins and their corresponding solutions:

<u>Problem 1: Dense or Tough Muffins</u>

- **Cause:** Overmixing the batter can lead to the development of gluten, resulting in dense or tough muffins.

- **Solution:** Gently fold the wet and dry ingredients together until just combined. Avoid overmixing to maintain a light and tender texture.

Problem 2: Muffins Stick to Liners

- **Cause:** Muffins sticking to paper liners can be due to the moisture content in the batter.

- **Solution:** Consider using non-stick cooking spray on the liners or greasing the muffin tin before placing the liners. Alternatively, you can let the muffins cool slightly before removing them from the liners.

Problem 3: Uneven Baking

- **Cause:** If the muffins are not baked evenly, it could be due to uneven distribution of batter or uneven oven temperature.

- <u>Solution:</u> Ensure that you fill each muffin cup with a similar amount of batter to ensure even baking. Also, use an oven thermometer to check and adjust your oven's temperature if necessary.

<u>Problem 4: Soggy Bottoms</u>

- Cause: Muffins having a soggy bottom might be caused by underbaking or excess moisture in the batter.

- Solution: Make sure to bake the muffins until a toothpick inserted into the center comes out clean. Additionally, avoid adding too much liquid to the batter.

<u>Problem 5: Muffins Collapse or Sink in the Middle</u>

- Cause: Muffins that collapse or sink in the middle after baking might have risen too quickly and then collapsed.

- **Solution:** Double-check your leavening agents (baking powder and baking soda) measurements. Also, avoid opening the oven door during the first half of baking, as rapid temperature changes can cause muffins to collapse.

Problem 6: Overly Browned Tops

- **Cause:** If the tops of the muffins are browning too quickly, it could be due to a higher oven temperature.

- **Solution:** Lower the oven temperature slightly or cover the muffins with aluminum foil during the latter part of baking to prevent excessive browning.

<u>Delicious Avocado Tomato Toast</u>

Avocado toast with tomato salsa is a delightful and nutritious culinary creation that has gained immense popularity in recent years. Combining the creamy richness of avocado with the vibrant freshness of tomato salsa, this dish offers a burst of flavors and textures that tantalize the taste buds.

At its core, avocado toast with tomato salsa is a harmonious marriage of two distinct elements. The velvety smoothness of ripe avocado is contrasted by the zesty, tangy notes of tomato salsa, resulting in a symphony of flavors that dance across the palate. The simplicity of the dish allows these key ingredients to shine, with each bite offering a satisfying blend of creamy, crunchy, and juicy components.

The preparation of this dish is relatively straightforward. A ripe avocado is mashed onto a slice of toasted bread, acting as a creamy base. The avocado not only imparts a rich taste but also provides a dose of healthy fats and essential nutrients. On top of the avocado, a generous serving of tomato salsa is piled, bringing a burst of color and freshness to the dish. The salsa, often made with diced tomatoes, onions, cilantro, lime juice, and a touch of spice, adds a zingy and vibrant character to the toast.

One of the defining features of avocado toast with tomato salsa is its versatility. The basic recipe can be easily customized to suit individual preferences and dietary restrictions. Additional toppings such as poached eggs, crumbled feta cheese, or a sprinkle of flax seeds can be added to enhance both the flavor profile and nutritional value. The dish can be enjoyed as a hearty breakfast, a light lunch, or even a satisfying snack.

Beyond its delectable taste, avocado toast with tomato salsa carries several health benefits. Avocado is known for its high content of monounsaturated fats, which are considered heart-healthy fats. Additionally, avocados are a great source of vitamins, minerals, and fiber. The tomato salsa complements this nutritional profile with its vitamin C content and antioxidants, contributing to overall well-being.

Avocado toast with tomato salsa is a culinary masterpiece that harmonizes contrasting flavors and textures to create a satisfying and nutritious dish. Its simplicity, adaptability, and health benefits have made it a staple on menus and breakfast tables around the world. Whether enjoyed as a leisurely brunch or a quick snack, this dish offers a delightful experience that is as pleasing to the palate as it is beneficial to the body.

Avocado Toast Recipe

Sure, here's a simple itemized process for preparing Avocado Toast with Tomato Salsa:

1. Gather Ingredients:

Ripe avocados

Bread slices (such as whole grain or sourdough)

Tomatoes

Red onion

Fresh cilantro

Lime juice

Salt and pepper

Optional: Red pepper flakes, feta cheese, poached egg

2. Make Tomato Salsa:

- Dice tomatoes and finely chop red onion.

- Chop fresh cilantro.

- In a bowl, combine tomatoes, red onion, and cilantro.

- Add a squeeze of lime juice and season with salt and pepper to taste.

- Optional: Add a pinch of red pepper flakes for some heat.

3. Prepare Avocado:

- Cut ripe avocados in half and remove the pits.

- Scoop the avocado flesh into a bowl.

- Mash the avocado with a fork until you reach your desired consistency.

- Add a squeeze of lime juice, salt, and pepper to taste.

4. Toast Bread:

- Toast the bread slices until they are golden brown and crispy.

5. Assemble the Avocado Toast:

- Spread the mashed avocado onto the toasted bread slices.

6. Top with Tomato Salsa:

- Spoon the prepared tomato salsa over the mashed avocado.

7. Optional Additions:

- If desired, crumble feta cheese over the top for added creaminess and flavor.

- You can also add a poached egg on top for extra protein and richness.

8. Serve:

- Serve the avocado toast with tomato salsa immediately while it's still fresh and the flavors are vibrant.

<u>Delicious Avocado Tomato Toast The problems and solutions</u>

Here are some potential problems that could arise while preparing Avocado Toast with Tomato Salsa, along with their solutions:

<u>Problem 1: Unripe Avocado:</u>

- If the avocados are not ripe, they will be difficult to mash and won't have the desired creamy texture.

Solution:

- Ensure you select ripe avocados that yield slightly to gentle pressure when squeezed. If your avocados are not ripe enough, you can place them in a paper bag at room temperature to speed up the ripening process.

<u>Problem 2: Overripe Avocado:</u>

- If the avocados are overripe, they might have a bitter taste and an unappetizing appearance.

Solution:

- Gently squeeze the avocados before cutting them open to check for overripeness. If the avocados are too soft and mushy, they may be overripe. Discard any portions that are brown or spoiled.

Problem 3: Soggy Toast:

- If the bread slices are not toasted properly, they might become soggy when topped with avocado and tomato salsa.

Solution:

- Toast the bread slices until they are golden brown and crispy. This will help maintain their texture even when topped with moist ingredients.

Problem 4: Inadequate Seasoning:

- Failing to season the avocado mash and tomato salsa properly can result in bland flavors.

Solution:

- Taste and adjust the seasoning of both the avocado mash and tomato salsa. Add enough salt, pepper, and lime juice to enhance the flavors.

Problem 5: Watery Salsa:

- If the tomato salsa becomes too watery, it can make the toast soggy.

Solution:

- After dicing the tomatoes, you can place them in a strainer for a few minutes to allow the excess liquid to drain. Alternatively, you can gently pat the diced tomatoes with a paper towel to remove excess moisture.

Problem 6: Ingredient Allergies or Preferences:

- Some individuals might have allergies or dietary preferences that require omitting certain ingredients.

Solution:

- Customize the recipe to suit individual preferences or dietary restrictions. For example, you can omit ingredients like onions or feta cheese if necessary.

By being mindful of these potential problems and their solutions, you can ensure a successful and enjoyable cooking experience while preparing Avocado Toast with Tomato Salsa.

Delightful Soups & Salads

In the realm of culinary delights, hearty soups, and salads stand as versatile champions, offering a symphony of flavors, textures, and nutrition. These two culinary genres have earned their place on menus worldwide, providing comfort and sustenance to people of all ages and palates. Let's delve into the world of hearty soups and salads, exploring their merits and popularity.

Hearty soups, often referred to as comfort in a bowl, warm both the body and soul. From creamy chowders to chunky stews, they boast an array of ingredients that come together harmoniously. A steaming bowl of chicken noodle soup or a rich tomato bisque on a chilly day evokes nostalgia and warmth. The key lies in the slow simmering of ingredients, allowing flavors to meld and intensify. Hearty soups are not only a culinary delight but also a nourishing choice, often packed with vegetables, proteins, and whole grains.

On the other hand, salads are a celebration of freshness and crunch. Ranging from simple garden salads to complex creations featuring a plethora of ingredients, salads are the epitome of culinary creativity. They offer a burst of color, a variety of textures, and an abundance of vitamins and minerals. A classic Caesar salad with crisp romaine lettuce, crunchy croutons, tangy dressing, and savory parmesan shavings is a timeless favorite. Salads are not confined to just greens; they can incorporate fruits, nuts, seeds, cheeses, and proteins, catering to every taste preference.

Beyond their sensory pleasures, both hearty soups and salads cater to various dietary needs. They can be adapted to vegetarian, vegan, gluten-free, and other dietary restrictions, making them inclusive options for diverse dining preferences. Additionally, the customizable nature of salads and the adaptability of soup recipes mean that they can suit different seasons and occasions.

In recent years, the culinary world has witnessed a renaissance in both hearty soups and salads. Chefs and home cooks alike experiment with unusual ingredients, unique flavor combinations, and innovative presentations, transforming these traditional dishes into contemporary works of art. The fusion of cultural influences and culinary techniques has led to the creation of soups and salads that transcend borders and redefine culinary boundaries.

In conclusion, hearty soups and salads are more than mere dishes; they are a testament to the versatility and creativity that the culinary world offers. Whether seeking comfort or vitality, traditional flavors, or modern twists, these dishes stand as delicious reminders of the joy that food can bring. As they continue to evolve with the times, hearty soups and salads remain beloved staples, nourishing both body and spirit with every spoonful and forkful.

<u>Various Delightful Soups & Salads</u>

In the realm of gastronomy, few dishes are as versatile and delightful as soups and salads. These culinary creations not only tantalize the taste buds but also provide a wholesome and nourishing experience. From the comforting warmth of a hearty soup to the refreshing crunch of a vibrant salad, the world of flavors they encompass is truly a treat for the senses.

Soups, with their steaming cauldrons of flavors, evoke feelings of comfort and nostalgia. Whether it's a classic chicken noodle soup that warms the soul on a chilly day or a creamy tomato bisque that soothes the palate, each spoonful carries a story of tradition and innovation. From chunky stews to velvety purees, soups showcase the ingenuity of combining diverse ingredients into harmonious symphonies of taste.

On the other hand, salads present a visual and gustatory feast with their colorful medleys of crisp vegetables, succulent fruits, and tantalizing dressings. The humble greens transform into gourmet delicacies when adorned with ingredients like crumbled feta, candied nuts, or grilled chicken. The play of textures and the dance of flavors in a well-crafted salad is a celebration of nature's bounty.

From the hearty minestrone to the delicate gazpacho, soups vary from region to region, offering a glimpse into the culinary heritage of different cultures. Similarly, salads adapt to local produce and preferences, giving rise to the Greek salad, the Thai mango salad, and the Caprese salad, each a testament to the art of fusion and creativity.

In a world where culinary trends continue to evolve, soups and salads remain timeless classics that cater to a wide range of dietary preferences and health-conscious choices. They provide a canvas for experimentation, allowing chefs and home cooks alike to blend flavors, textures, and colors in ways that surprise and delight.

So, whether you're sipping on a steaming bowl of clam chowder or indulging in a crisp arugula and berry salad, remember that behind these simple yet exquisite dishes lies a world of culinary craftsmanship that never ceases to amaze and satisfy.

An itemized breakdown of various types of hearty soups reads as follows:

A. **<u>Hearty Soups:</u>**

1. **Chowders:** Creamy soups are often made with seafood (clam chowder, corn chowder) or vegetables (potato chowder).

2. **Stews:** Thick and substantial soups with chunks of meat (beef stew, lamb stew) and vegetables.

3. **Minestrone:** An Italian vegetable soup often featuring pasta or rice.

4. **Lentil Soup:** Made from lentils, this soup is protein-rich and comes in various regional variations.

5. **Chicken Noodle Soup:** Classic comfort food with chicken, noodles, and vegetables in a flavorful broth.

6. Tomato Soup: Smooth and velvety soup made from tomatoes, often served with bread or crackers.

7. Gumbo: A spicy Creole soup with a mix of meats, vegetables, and rice.

8. French Onion Soup: Featuring caramelized onions, topped with melted cheese and bread.

9. Bean Soup: Varieties like black bean soup, split pea soup, and white bean soup offer diverse flavors.

10. Borscht: A beet-based soup often served cold and originating from Eastern Europe.

B. **Hearty Salads:**

1. Cobb Salad: A salad with mixed greens, bacon, avocado, chicken, eggs, tomatoes, and blue cheese.

2. Caesar Salad: Romaine lettuce, croutons, parmesan cheese, and Caesar dressing.

3. Nicoise Salad: A French salad with tuna, green beans, potatoes, olives, and hard-boiled eggs.

4. Greek Salad: Featuring tomatoes, cucumbers, olives, feta cheese, onions, and Greek dressing.

5. Waldorf Salad: A fruity salad with apples, grapes, celery, walnuts, and mayonnaise dressing.

6. Caprese Salad: Layers of tomato, mozzarella, and basil drizzled with olive oil and balsamic vinegar.

7. <u>Asian Chicken Salad</u>: Mixed greens, grilled chicken, mandarin oranges, almonds, and sesame dressing.

8. <u>Spinach Salad</u>: Spinach leaves with toppings like bacon, eggs, mushrooms, and warm dressing.

9. <u>Taco Salad:</u> A Tex-Mex creation with ground meat, lettuce, tomatoes, cheese, and tortilla chips.

10. <u>Fruit Salad</u>: A medley of fresh fruits, sometimes with added herbs, dressings, or yogurt.

This is a glimpse into the rich array of options within hearty soups and salads. The culinary world is vast and ever-evolving, offering a limitless combination of ingredients and flavors for these beloved dishes.

Lentil and Vegetable Soup

Lentil and vegetable soup stands as a testament to the perfect fusion of nutrition and comfort. This hearty dish combines the earthy richness of lentils with the vibrant flavors of assorted vegetables, resulting in a wholesome and satisfying meal that nourishes both body and soul.

At its core, lentil and vegetable soup encapsulates a harmony of tastes and textures. The humble lentils, rich in protein and fiber, provide a hearty base that promotes satiety and supports digestive health. As they simmer in the broth, they absorb the surrounding flavors, creating a broth that's not only delicious but also full of essential nutrients.

The medley of vegetables that grace this soup lends color, crunch, and a range of vitamins to the mix. Carrots offer sweetness and beta-carotene, while celery brings a hint of freshness and antioxidants. The versatility of this dish allows for personal preferences to shine, with ingredients like spinach, zucchini, or bell peppers adding unique dimensions to the final creation.

Preparing lentil and vegetable soup is not only about the end result but also the journey. Chopping, sautéing, and simmering the ingredients gradually releases their aromas, filling the kitchen with a comforting fragrance that evokes memories of home-cooked meals. As each ingredient is carefully added to the pot, the anticipation grows, leading to the reward of a warm bowl of nourishment.

This soup is not just a culinary delight; it's a well-rounded nutritional package. Its blend of protein, fiber, vitamins, and minerals supports a balanced diet and aids in maintaining overall well-being. Whether enjoyed as a light lunch or a hearty dinner, lentil and vegetable soup is a guilt-free indulgence that leaves one feeling satisfied and energized.

Lentil and vegetable soup is a testament to the beauty of simple, wholesome ingredients coming together to create a symphony of flavors and nourishment. It warms the body and soul, inviting comfort and satisfaction with every spoonful. As you savor each bite, remember that this dish is more than just a meal; it's a celebration of nature's bounty and the art of culinary craftsmanship.

Lentil and Vegetable Soup Prep

Cooking times and ingredient quantities may vary based on your preferences, so feel free to adjust as needed. Be careful with the quantity of ingredients you are about to use to prevent setbacks.

A step-by-step process for preparing Lentil and Vegetable Soup:

1. Gather Ingredients:

Collect red or green lentils, a variety of vegetables (such as carrots, celery, onions, and tomatoes), garlic, vegetable broth or water, olive oil, and seasonings (like salt, pepper, and herbs).

2. Prep Vegetables:

Wash, peel, and chop the vegetables into bite-sized pieces.

3. Rinse Lentils:

Thoroughly rinse the lentils in cold water and drain.

4. Sauté Aromatics:

In a large pot, heat olive oil and sauté chopped onions, garlic, and any other aromatic vegetables until they're softened and fragrant.

5. Add Vegetables:

Add the chopped vegetables to the pot and sauté for a few more minutes until they start to soften.

6. Add Lentils:

Incorporate the rinsed lentils into the pot and stir to combine.

7. Pour in Liquid:

Pour in vegetable broth or water, covering the lentils and vegetables. Adjust the liquid amount based on your desired soup consistency.

8. Season and Simmer:

Add salt, pepper, and any desired herbs (such as thyme, bay leaves, or rosemary). Bring the soup to a boil, then reduce the heat to a simmer. Cover the pot and let it cook until the lentils and vegetables are tender, usually around 20-30 minutes.

9. Check Seasoning:

Taste the soup and adjust the seasoning if needed. You can also add more liquid if the soup is too thick.

10. Serve and Enjoy:

Once the soup is cooked to your liking, remove any bay leaves if used. Serve the lentil and vegetable soup hot, and consider garnishing with fresh herbs or a drizzle of olive oil.

11. Optional Blending:

If you prefer a creamier texture, you can use an immersion blender to partially blend the soup while still leaving some chunks for texture.

12. Storage:

Allow the soup to cool before storing any leftovers in an airtight container in the refrigerator. It can stay fresh for a few days.

Enjoy your homemade Lentil and Vegetable Soup!

<u>Lentil and Vegetable Soup Problems and solutions</u>

Cooking is a creative process, and adapting to unexpected challenges is part of the fun. Don't hesitate to experiment and make adjustments as you go along to ensure your Lentil and Vegetable Soup turns out delicious and satisfying.

Now, let's go into the problems you might encounter while preparing Lentil and Vegetable Soup, along with their corresponding solutions:

<u>Problem 1: Overcooking Lentils and Vegetables</u>

Solution: Keep a close eye on the cooking time and texture. Lentils can become mushy if overcooked, so check for doneness by tasting them periodically. If they're soft but not mushy, remove the soup from heat.

Problem 2: Insufficient Seasoning

Solution: Taste the soup before serving and adjust the seasoning as needed. Add more salt, pepper, or herbs to enhance the flavor. Remember to season in small increments and taste after each addition.

Problem 3: Soup Too Thick or Thin

Solution: If the soup is too thick, add more vegetable broth, water, or even a bit of tomato sauce to achieve your desired consistency. If it's too thin, you can let it simmer uncovered for a bit longer to reduce the liquid.

Problem 4: Burnt Aromatics

Solution: Be cautious while sautéing onions, garlic, and other aromatic vegetables. Stir them frequently and adjust the heat if necessary to prevent burning. If you do encounter burnt bits, transfer the soup to a clean pot, leaving the burnt parts behind.

Problem 5: Unbalanced Flavors

Solution: If the flavors aren't coming together as you'd like, consider adding a splash of vinegar (such as red wine vinegar) or a squeeze of lemon juice to brighten the taste. A touch of sweetness from a small amount of sugar or honey can also help balance flavors.

Problem 6: Too Salty

Solution: If you accidentally make the soup too salty, you can balance it out by adding more unsalted vegetable broth or water. You can also add a starchy ingredient like chopped potatoes or cooked rice to help absorb excess salt.

Problem 7: Not Enough Time

Solution: If you're short on time, you can use pre-chopped or frozen vegetables to save on prep. Opt for pre-cooked lentils or canned lentils, which will significantly reduce the cooking time. Just be sure to adjust the liquid and cooking time accordingly.

Problem 8: Dietary Restrictions

Solution: If you have dietary restrictions or preferences, you can easily adapt the recipe. For example, use gluten-free vegetable broth for a gluten-free version, or swap out certain vegetables based on your taste and dietary needs.

Chickpea Salad with Lemon-Tahini Dressing

Eating healthy doesn't mean compromising on flavor, and a perfect example of this is the delightful Chickpea Salad with Lemon-Tahini Dressing. This vibrant and nutritious dish brings together the earthy goodness of chickpeas with the tangy zest of lemon and the creamy richness of tahini. It's a medley of textures and flavors that will leave your taste buds dancing.

To start, gather a can of chickpeas (garbanzo beans) or cook them from scratch if you prefer. Rinse and drain them well to remove excess starch. In a mixing bowl, combine the chickpeas with diced colorful bell peppers, cucumbers, cherry tomatoes, red onions, and chopped fresh parsley. This array of vegetables not only adds a burst of colors to the salad but also contributes a variety of nutrients.

The dressing is where the magic happens. In a separate bowl, whisk together tahini, freshly squeezed lemon juice, minced garlic, a touch of olive oil, and a pinch of salt and pepper. Adjust the ratios to your preference – more tahini for creaminess, more lemon for tanginess. Once the dressing is well combined, drizzle it over the chickpea and vegetable mixture.

Now comes the fun part – tossing everything together. The dressing coats the chickpeas and veggies, binding them together in a harmonious blend. The nutty flavor of tahini complements the bright acidity of lemon, while the garlic adds a gentle kick.

For added depth and texture, you can sprinkle toasted sesame seeds or chopped nuts like almonds or walnuts on top. These ingredients provide a satisfying crunch that contrasts beautifully with the softer components of the salad.

Chill the Chickpea Salad with Lemon-Tahini Dressing in the refrigerator for about half an hour before serving. This allows the flavors to meld and develop, resulting in a more delightful eating experience. It's a refreshing dish that can be enjoyed on its own as a light lunch or dinner, or served as a side to grilled chicken, fish, or pita bread.

Not only is this salad a treat for your taste buds, but it's also a powerhouse of nutrients. Chickpeas are rich in protein, fiber, and various vitamins and minerals, while the vegetables provide a spectrum of vitamins and antioxidants. The lemon-tahini dressing contributes healthy fats and a burst of zesty freshness.

Chickpea Salad with Lemon-Tahini Dressing is a culinary masterpiece that marries health and flavor effortlessly. It's a versatile dish that suits various occasions and dietary preferences, making it a must-try recipe for anyone looking to enjoy a nutritious and delicious meal.

Chickpea Salad with Lemon-Tahini Prep

Here, you need to be aware that quantities can be adjusted based on your preference and the number of servings needed.

1. Gather Ingredients:

- 2 cans of chickpeas (15 oz each)
- 1 cucumber, diced
- 1 red bell pepper, diced
- 1/2 red onion, finely chopped
- 1 cup cherry tomatoes, halved
- 1/4 cup fresh parsley, chopped
- 1/4 cup feta cheese, crumbled
- 1/4 cup Kalamata olives, pitted and chopped

2. Make Lemon-Tahini Dressing:

- In a bowl, whisk together 1/4 cup tahini, 3 tablespoons lemon juice, 2 tablespoons olive oil, 1 minced garlic clove, 1 teaspoon honey, and salt and pepper to taste. Adjust the seasoning according to your preference.

3. Prepare Chickpeas:

- Drain and rinse the chickpeas from the cans. Pat them dry with a paper towel.

4. Combine Ingredients:

- In a large bowl, combine the chickpeas, diced cucumber, diced red bell pepper, finely chopped red onion, halved cherry tomatoes, and chopped parsley.

5. Add Dressing:

- Pour the lemon-tahini dressing over the salad and gently toss everything together until well combined.

6. Add Toppings:

- Sprinkle crumbled feta cheese and chopped Kalamata olives on top of the salad.

7. Chill and Serve:

- Cover the salad and let it chill in the refrigerator for about 30 minutes to allow the flavors to meld together.

8. Serve:

- Once chilled, give the salad a final toss before serving. You can serve it as a side dish or a light meal on its own.

Chickpea Salad with Lemon-Tahini Prep The problems and solutions

There are some potential problems you might encounter while preparing Chickpea Salad with Lemon-Tahini Dressing, along with their solutions:

Problem 1: Overly Thick Dressing

- **Solution:** If your Lemon-Tahini Dressing turns out too thick, gradually add a bit more lemon juice or water while whisking until you achieve the desired consistency.

Problem 2: Bland Salad

- **Solution:** To enhance the flavors of the salad, make sure to season each component well with salt and pepper. Additionally, you can experiment with adding more fresh herbs, such as mint or basil, for added depth of flavor.

Problem 3: Watery Salad

- **Solution:** To prevent a watery salad, make sure to drain and pat dry the chickpeas before combining them with the other ingredients. Also, consider using a slotted spoon to serve the salad, which will help drain excess moisture.

Problem 4: Inconsistent Dressing Distribution

- **Solution:** When adding the Lemon-Tahini Dressing to the salad, pour it over the ingredients in portions and toss gently after each addition. This will help distribute the dressing evenly and ensure that all parts of the salad are coated.

<u>Problem 5: Soggy Vegetables</u>

- **Solution:** To avoid soggy vegetables, dice them into uniform sizes. If you're making the salad in advance, you can keep the chopped vegetables and dressing separate until you're ready to serve, then combine them just before serving.

Problem 6: Dietary Restrictions

- **Solution:** If you or your guests have dietary restrictions, such as dairy or gluten sensitivities, consider omitting the feta cheese or using a dairy-free alternative. Additionally, ensure that all ingredients, including the tahini and honey, align with the dietary needs.

Problem 7: Adjusting Quantities

- **Solution:** The quantities provided in the recipe are approximate and can be adjusted based on your preferences and the number of servings you need. Feel free to scale up or down according to your requirements.

Be aware that cooking is a creative process, and it's okay to experiment and make adjustments along the way to suit your taste and needs.

Quinoa and Spinach Salad

This vibrant salad is not only visually appealing but also a powerhouse of nutrients, making it a popular choice among health-conscious individuals. Quinoa and spinach salad is a delightful and nutritious dish that brings together the wholesome goodness of quinoa and the refreshing flavors of spinach.

At the heart of this salad is quinoa, a versatile and protein-rich grain that is considered a complete protein source, containing all nine essential amino acids. Quinoa's nutty flavor and slightly crunchy texture complement the tender leaves of spinach perfectly. Spinach, known for its high iron and vitamin content, adds a burst of color and a mild earthy taste to the dish.

To create this salad, start by cooking quinoa according to the package instructions, usually requiring a quick rinse and simmering. Once cooked, allow it to cool.

Meanwhile, prepare the spinach by washing and drying the leaves thoroughly. Feel free to tear them into bite-sized pieces to ensure an even distribution in the salad.

For added variety and flavor, you can incorporate an assortment of colorful vegetables such as cherry tomatoes, diced bell peppers, grated carrots, and cucumber slices. These ingredients not only enhance the salad's appearance but also contribute to its nutritional profile.

To bring all the components together, prepare a light and tangy vinaigrette. A simple combination of olive oil, lemon juice, minced garlic, salt, and pepper can provide a refreshing balance to the earthy notes of quinoa and spinach.

Combine the cooled quinoa, spinach, and chopped vegetables in a large bowl. Drizzle the vinaigrette over the salad and gently toss everything together until well-coated. This allows the flavors to meld and ensures every bite is bursting with taste.

The quinoa and spinach salad is not only an excellent choice for a light lunch or dinner but also a versatile side dish that can be served alongside grilled proteins, roasted vegetables, or even as a topping for warm pita bread. Its combination of textures, flavors, and nutritional benefits make it a go-to option for those seeking a well-rounded and satisfying meal.

In conclusion, the quinoa and spinach salad is a testament to the harmony between nutritious ingredients and culinary creativity. Its ability to please both the palate and the body makes it a staple in modern healthy eating, offering a delightful experience with every forkful.

Quinoa Spinach Salad Recipe

An itemized process for preparing a Quinoa and Spinach Salad are as follows:

Quinoa

1. Ingredients:

- 1 cup quinoa

- 2 cups water or vegetable broth

- 2 cups fresh spinach leaves, washed and chopped

- 1 cup cherry tomatoes, halved

- 1/2 cup red onion, finely chopped

- 1/4 cup feta cheese, crumbled

- 1/4 cup toasted pine nuts

- 2 tablespoons olive oil

- 2 tablespoons lemon juice

- Salt and pepper to taste

Spinach Quinoa salad

2. Cook Quinoa:

- Rinse the quinoa under cold water.

- In a saucepan, combine quinoa and water (or vegetable broth) and bring to a boil.

- Reduce heat to low, cover, and simmer for about 15 minutes or until quinoa is cooked and water is absorbed.

- Remove from heat, fluff with a fork, and let it cool slightly.

3. Prepare Dressing:

- In a small bowl, whisk together olive oil, lemon juice, salt, and pepper to create the dressing.

4. Combine Ingredients:

- In a large mixing bowl, combine the cooked quinoa, chopped spinach, halved cherry tomatoes, finely chopped red onion, crumbled feta cheese, and toasted pine nuts.

5. Add Dressing:

- Pour the prepared dressing over the quinoa and vegetable mixture.

6. Toss and Adjust Seasoning:

- Gently toss all the ingredients together to evenly coat them with the dressing.

- Taste and adjust seasoning with more salt, pepper, or lemon juice if needed.

7. Serve:

- Transfer the quinoa and spinach salad to serving plates or bowls.

8. Optional Garnish:

- You can add some additional crumbled feta cheese or toasted pine nuts on top for extra flavor and texture.

9. Enjoy:

- Serve the quinoa and spinach salad immediately as a nutritious and flavorful meal.

Ingredient quantities are adjustable to match your preferences and the number of servings you need.

<u>Problems and Solutions to Quinoa Spinach Salad Recipe</u>

Let's highlight some potential problems that might arise during the preparation of Quinoa and Spinach Salad and provide solutions for each:

<u>Problem 1: Overcooked or Undercooked Quinoa</u>

- Solution: Make sure to follow the cooking instructions and recommended water-to-quinoa ratio. If it's undercooked, add a bit more liquid and continue cooking. If it's overcooked, let it sit uncovered to cool and dry out a bit before using.

Problem 2: Bland Salad

- **Solution:** Adjust the seasoning of the dressing by adding more salt, pepper, or lemon juice to taste. You can also consider adding herbs like chopped fresh basil or parsley for added flavor.

Problem 3: Soggy Spinach

- **Solution:** Ensure that the spinach leaves are thoroughly washed and dried before chopping and adding to the salad. You can use a salad spinner or pat them dry with a clean kitchen towel.

Problem 4: Watery Dressing

- **Solution:** If the dressing ends up too watery, adjust the ratios by adding a bit more olive oil or lemon juice. You can also whisk in a teaspoon of Dijon mustard to help emulsify and thicken the dressing.

Problem 5: Ingredient Imbalance

- **Solution:** While adjusting the quantities based on your preferences is fine, make sure not to overwhelm the salad with one ingredient. Aim for a balanced mix of quinoa, spinach, tomatoes, onion, cheese, and nuts for the best flavor and texture.

Problem 6: Nut Allergies

- **Solution:** If you or someone you're serving the salad to has nut allergies, omit the pine nuts or replace them with a safe alternative like toasted sunflower seeds or pumpkin seeds.

Problem 7: Skipping the Cooling Step

- **Solution:** Allowing the cooked quinoa to cool slightly before combining it with the other ingredients prevents wilting of the spinach and helps the flavors meld together better.

Problem 8: Not Adjusting the Recipe for Dietary Restrictions

- **Solution:** If you have dietary restrictions, such as dairy-free or vegan, choose a dairy-free cheese alternative or omit the cheese altogether. Additionally, ensure that all the ingredients you use align with your dietary needs.

By being aware of these potential issues and applying the suggested solutions, you'll be better equipped to prepare a delicious and successful Quinoa and Spinach Salad.

<u>Satisfying Main Dishes</u>

A well-prepared main dish is the centerpiece of any meal, providing a hearty and satisfying experience that leaves taste buds delighted and appetites fulfilled. Whether it's a family dinner or a special occasion, the choice of a main dish can define the entire dining experience. From comfort foods to gourmet creations, there's an array of options to suit various palates and preferences.

One beloved category of satisfying main dishes is comfort food classics. These dishes evoke feelings of nostalgia and warmth, often featuring familiar ingredients prepared in delightful ways. Think of dishes like macaroni and cheese, pot roast, or meatloaf – they offer a sense of familiarity that brings people together around the table.

For those seeking a more adventurous culinary journey, gourmet main dishes offer a delightful exploration of flavors and textures. From beautifully plated seafood dishes to expertly grilled steaks, these creations cater to the discerning palate. Gourmet dishes often incorporate a fusion of global influences, combining ingredients and techniques from different cuisines to create something truly unique.

Vegetarian and vegan main dishes have also gained popularity, showcasing the versatility of plant-based ingredients. Dishes like stuffed bell peppers, mushroom risotto, or lentil curry provide both nourishment and satisfaction without relying on animal products. These options not only offer a healthier alternative but also cater to individuals with dietary restrictions.

In recent years, there's been a surge in the popularity of bowl-based main dishes. Burrito bowls, poke bowls, and grain bowls allow for customization and balance.

These dishes typically feature a variety of proteins, vegetables, grains, and flavorful sauces, providing a harmonious blend of textures and tastes in every bite.

Ultimately, the choice of a satisfying main dish depends on personal preferences and the occasion. The art of preparing and enjoying a main dish goes beyond mere sustenance – it's a chance to indulge the senses, share stories, and create lasting memories. So whether you're savoring a timeless comfort food or indulging in a gourmet masterpiece, the main dish remains the heart of a truly satisfying culinary experience.

<u>Zucchini Noodles with Pesto</u>

Zucchini Noodles with Pesto is a delicious and healthy dish that has gained popularity as a low-carb alternative to traditional pasta. Zucchini noodles, also known as "zoodles," are created by spiralizing fresh zucchini into thin strands that resemble spaghetti. These zoodles provide a light and refreshing base for various sauces, with pesto being a standout choice.

Pesto is a classic Italian sauce made from a combination of fresh basil, pine nuts, garlic, Parmesan cheese, and olive oil. The ingredients are blended together to create a vibrant green sauce that's full of flavor. When paired with zucchini noodles, pesto adds a burst of herbaceous and nutty taste that complements the mild, slightly sweet flavor of the zucchini.

To make Zucchini Noodles with Pesto, start by spiralizing the zucchini using a spiralizer or a julienne peeler. You can then lightly sauté the zoodles in a pan with a touch of olive oil for a few minutes, just until they are slightly softened. Be careful not to overcook them, as zucchini noodles can become mushy if cooked for too long.

Next, toss the sautéed zoodles with the freshly prepared pesto sauce. You can adjust the amount of pesto according to your taste preferences. The pesto will coat the zucchini noodles evenly, providing a burst of vibrant color and a delightful aroma.

Feel free to customize this dish by adding additional ingredients. Cherry tomatoes, roasted red peppers, or grilled chicken are some great options to enhance both the flavor and visual appeal of the dish. You can also sprinkle some extra grated Parmesan cheese or toasted pine nuts on top for added texture and richness.

Zucchini Noodles with Pesto is not only a flavorful and satisfying meal, but it's also a fantastic way to incorporate more vegetables into your diet. It's particularly popular among individuals who are following a low-carb or gluten-free lifestyle. This dish is not only delicious but also showcases the versatility of zucchini and the timeless appeal of pesto sauce.

Zucchini Noodles with Pesto Prep

1. Ingredients:

- 2 medium zucchinis

- 1/2 cup of fresh basil leaves

- 1/4 cup of pine nuts

- 1/4 cup of grated Parmesan cheese

- 1 clove of garlic

- 1/3 cup of extra virgin olive oil

- Salt and pepper to taste

2. Prepare the Zucchini Noodles:

- Wash and dry the zucchinis.

- Using a spiralizer or a vegetable peeler, cut the zucchinis into long, thin noodle-like strips. Place them in a colander, sprinkle with a little salt, and let them sit for about 15 minutes to release excess moisture. Pat dry with paper towels.

3. Make the Pesto:

- In a food processor, combine the fresh basil, pine nuts, grated Parmesan cheese, and garlic clove.

- Pulse the mixture until coarsely chopped.

- While the food processor is running, gradually pour in the olive oil in a steady stream until the mixture becomes smooth and well combined.

- Season with salt and pepper to taste.

4. Assemble the Dish:

- In a large bowl, toss the zucchini noodles with the freshly prepared pesto until the noodles are well coated.

5. Serve:

- Divide the zucchini noodles with pesto among serving plates.

- Optionally, you can garnish with extra grated Parmesan cheese and a few extra basil leaves.

6. Enjoy:

- Serve the zucchini noodles with pesto as a light and flavorful meal. It can be served cold or slightly warmed.

Zucchini Noodles with Pesto Prep Problems and Solutions

These are some potential problems you might encounter while preparing Zucchini Noodles with Pesto, along with their solutions:

Problem 1: Excess Moisture in Zucchini Noodles

- When making zucchini noodles, they might release excess moisture, making the dish watery.

Solution:

- Sprinkle the zucchini noodles with salt and let them sit in a colander for about 15 minutes before patting them dry with paper towels. This will help remove excess moisture and prevent the dish from becoming too watery.

Problem 2: Pesto Too Thick or Thin

- The pesto might turn out too thick or too thin, affecting the consistency of the dish.

Solution:

- If the pesto is too thick, gradually add a bit more olive oil while blending until you achieve the desired consistency.
- If the pesto is too thin, you can add more basil leaves, pine nuts, or grated Parmesan cheese to thicken it.

Problem 3: Overpowering Garlic Flavor

- Adding too much garlic can result in an overpowering flavor that might dominate the dish.

Solution:

- Use a single clove of garlic and adjust the quantity based on your preference. You can start with half a clove if you're concerned about the garlic flavor being too strong.

Problem 4: Unbalanced Flavors

- The flavors of the pesto might not be well balanced, leading to a bland or overly strong taste.

Solution:

- Taste the pesto as you prepare it and adjust the amounts of basil, pine nuts, cheese, olive oil, salt, and pepper accordingly to achieve a well-balanced flavor profile.

Problem 5: Allergic Reactions or Dietary Restrictions

- Some individuals may have allergies to nuts or dairy products, which are common ingredients in traditional pesto.

Solution:

- To accommodate allergies or dietary restrictions, consider using alternatives such as sunflower seeds or nutritional yeast instead of pine nuts and cheese, respectively.

Problem 6: Spiralizing Difficulties

- Spiralizing the zucchinis can be challenging, especially if you don't have the right equipment.

Solution:

- If you don't have a spiralizer, you can use a vegetable peeler to create wide, flat ribbons of zucchini. Alternatively, you can purchase pre-spiralized zucchini from some grocery stores.

Black Bean Tacos with Mango Salsa

Tacos have always been a beloved dish, known for their versatility and ability to bring together various flavors and textures. One such delightful variation is the Black Bean Tacos with Mango Salsa. This fusion of savory black beans and sweet, tangy mango salsa creates a culinary experience that tantalizes the taste buds and satisfies the senses.

At the heart of these tacos lies the protein-rich black beans, which not only provide a hearty base but also contribute to a balanced diet. Their creamy texture and earthy taste blend seamlessly with the vibrant mango salsa, which is a symphony of fresh mango chunks, red onions, cilantro, lime juice, and a hint of heat from jalapenos.

The contrasting textures in this dish play a crucial role in elevating its appeal. The softness of the black beans is contrasted by the crunch of the taco shell, creating a delightful interplay of sensations with every bite. The juiciness of the mango salsa complements the beans and adds a burst of tropical sweetness, making the experience truly captivating.

What makes this dish truly special is the amalgamation of flavors. The natural sweetness of the mango balances the savory notes of the beans, while the zing from the lime juice and the freshness of the cilantro brighten up the overall profile. This fusion showcases the beauty of combining seemingly disparate elements into a harmonious symphony of taste.

Moreover, the Black Bean Tacos with Mango Salsa cater to a wide range of dietary preferences. They are not only vegetarian but can also be made vegan by using plant-based taco shells and ensuring all the ingredients in the salsa are animal product-free. This inclusivity adds to the dish's charm, making it a choice that can be relished by a diverse audience.

Black Bean Tacos with Mango Salsa exemplify the magic that happens when culinary traditions collide. This fusion dish marries the heartiness of black beans with the sweetness of mango salsa, creating a medley of flavors and textures that dance on the palate. Whether enjoyed as a main course or served at gatherings, these tacos are a testament to the limitless possibilities of gastronomy.

Black Bean Tacos with Mango Salsa Prep

Here is basic outline of the process for preparing "Black Bean Tacos with Mango Salsa":

Ingredients:

- 1 can of black beans (15 oz)

- 1 cup diced mango

- 1/4 cup diced red onion

- 1/4 cup chopped cilantro

- 1 lime (juiced)

- 1 teaspoon cumin

- 1 teaspoon chili powder

- Salt and pepper to taste

- 8 small corn tortillas

- Optional toppings: sliced avocado, shredded lettuce, crumbled feta cheese

Instructions:

1. Prepare the Mango Salsa:

- In a bowl, combine the diced mango, red onion, chopped cilantro, and lime juice.

- Mix well and season with salt and pepper to taste.

- Set aside in the refrigerator to let the flavors meld.

2. Cook the Black Beans:

- Drain and rinse the canned black beans.

- In a saucepan, heat a small amount of oil over medium heat.

- Add the black beans, cumin, and chili powder.

- Cook for a few minutes until the beans are heated through and the spices are fragrant.

- Use a fork to lightly mash some of the beans. This will help create a nice texture for the tacos.

3. Warm the Tortillas:

- Heat the corn tortillas in a dry skillet or directly over a gas flame for a few seconds on each side until they are warm and pliable.

4. Assemble the Tacos:

- Place a spoonful of the black bean mixture onto each tortilla.

- Top with a generous spoonful of the mango salsa.

- Add any optional toppings you like, such as sliced avocado, shredded lettuce, or crumbled feta cheese.

5. Serve:

- Arrange the assembled tacos on a serving platter.

- Serve immediately, and enjoy your delicious Black Bean Tacos with Mango Salsa!

Black Bean Tacos with Mango Salsa Probs and Solutions

Some potential problems might arise while preparing Black Bean Tacos with Mango Salsa, along with their corresponding solutions:

Problem 1: Overly salty salsa

- If the mango salsa turns out too salty:

Solution: Taste and adjust the seasoning. You can add more diced mango or a squeeze of lime juice to balance out the saltiness.

Problem 2: Dry or flavorless beans

- If the black bean mixture is too dry or lacks flavor:

Solution: Add a splash of vegetable broth or water to the black bean mixture to add moisture and enhance the flavor. You can also adjust the seasoning by adding more cumin and chili powder.

Problem 3: Tortillas are difficult to work with

- If the corn tortillas are cracking or breaking when you try to fold them:

Solution: Heat the tortillas properly until they are soft and pliable. You can do this by briefly warming them in a skillet or over an open flame. Additionally, consider using two tortillas per taco to make them more sturdy.

Problem 4: Mango salsa is too tangy

- If the mango salsa is too tangy from the lime juice:

Solution: Balance out the tanginess by adding a bit more diced mango or a pinch of sugar to the salsa.

Problem 5: Tacos are falling apart

- If the tacos are falling apart when you try to eat them:

Solution: Make sure to not overfill the tacos. Start with a spoonful of the black bean mixture and then layer the mango salsa and other toppings. If the tortillas are too delicate, you can also double them up to make them sturdier.

Problem 6: Tacos are too bland

- If the overall flavor of the tacos is too bland:

Solution: Be sure to season each component well. Add more cumin, chili powder, or salt as needed. You can also consider adding some extra toppings like sliced jalapeños or a drizzle of hot sauce for added flavor.

Mushroom and Spinach Stir-Fry

Mushroom and spinach stir-fry is a delightful and nutritious dish that brings together the earthy flavors of mushrooms and the vibrant freshness of spinach. This simple yet flavorful recipe is a perfect choice for those seeking a quick and healthy meal option.

To begin, gather the ingredients: fresh mushrooms (such as button or cremini), fresh spinach leaves, garlic, onions, soy sauce, and your choice of cooking oil. Start by cleaning and slicing the mushrooms into thin pieces. Next, wash and pat dry the spinach leaves, removing any tough stems.

In a heated pan, add a dash of cooking oil and sauté finely chopped garlic and onions until they turn translucent. Then, add the sliced mushrooms and let them cook until they release their moisture and start to brown. The aroma that fills the kitchen at this stage is truly enticing.

Once the mushrooms are nicely cooked, it's time to add the fresh spinach leaves. The spinach will wilt quickly, so it's essential to keep stirring gently. As the leaves begin to wilt, drizzle in some soy sauce for flavor and a touch of saltiness.

In just a few minutes, the spinach will be perfectly cooked, retaining its vibrant green color. The mushrooms and spinach will have absorbed the flavors of the garlic, onions, and soy sauce, creating a harmonious blend of tastes.

This mushroom and spinach stir-fry can be served as a standalone dish or paired with steamed rice, quinoa, or noodles. For those who enjoy a bit of heat, a sprinkle of red pepper flakes or a dash of hot sauce can add an exciting kick.

Not only does this dish tantalize your taste buds, but it's also a nutritional powerhouse. Spinach is rich in vitamins and minerals, while mushrooms offer a good dose of protein and immune-boosting properties.

The mushroom and spinach stir-fry is a testament to the beauty of simplicity in cooking. With just a handful of ingredients and minimal effort, you can create a wholesome and flavorful meal that satisfies both the palate and the body. So, whether you're a seasoned chef or a beginner in the kitchen, this dish is a must-try for its ease, taste, and nutritional value.

Mushroom and Spinach Stir-Fry Prep

An itemized process for preparing Mushroom and Spinach Stir-Fry is as follows:

Ingredients:

- 250g mushrooms, sliced

- 200g spinach, washed and chopped

- 1 tablespoon olive oil

- 2 cloves garlic, minced

- 1 teaspoon ginger, minced

- 1 tablespoon soy sauce

- 1/2 teaspoon sesame oil

- Salt and pepper to taste

- Optional: red pepper flakes for some heat

<u>Instructions:</u>

1. Heat the olive oil in a large pan over medium-high heat.

2. Add the minced garlic and ginger. Sauté for about 30 seconds until fragrant.

3. Add the sliced mushrooms and cook for 3-4 minutes until they start to soften and release their moisture.

4. Stir in the chopped spinach and cook for an additional 2-3 minutes until wilted.

5. Drizzle in the soy sauce and sesame oil, and give everything a good stir to combine.

6. Season with salt, pepper, and red pepper flakes if using. Adjust seasoning to taste.

7. Continue to cook for another 1-2 minutes, allowing the flavors to meld together.

8. Remove from heat and serve the Mushroom and Spinach Stir-fry immediately as a side dish or overcooked rice or noodles.

Mushroom and Spinach Stir-Fry Challenges and Solutions

These are challenges that you might encounter while preparing Mushroom and Spinach Stir-Fry, along with possible solutions as follows:

Challenges:

1. Mushroom Moisture: Mushrooms release a lot of moisture when cooked, which can lead to a soggy stir-fry.

Solution: To prevent this, make sure the pan is hot before adding the mushrooms. Cook them in batches if necessary, allowing space between slices for moisture to evaporate. High heat will help evaporate excess moisture.

2. Overcooking Spinach: Spinach can quickly go from fresh to wilted and overcooked.

Solution: Add spinach towards the end of cooking to prevent overcooking. Stir it in for just a couple of minutes until it wilts, and then remove from heat promptly.

3. Flavor Balance: Achieving the right balance of flavors, especially between the soy sauce and sesame oil, can be tricky.

Solution: Start with a small amount of soy sauce and sesame oil, and taste as you go. You can always add more, but you can't take it away. Remember that you can adjust the seasoning at the end.

4. Texture Concerns: Overcooking mushrooms can result in a rubbery texture, and if spinach is overcooked, it can become mushy.

Solution: Keep a close eye on the cooking time and use high heat for mushrooms to achieve a nice sear. Aim for vibrant green spinach, not a mushy texture.

5. Garlic and Ginger Burning: Minced garlic and ginger can burn quickly, resulting in a bitter taste.

Solution: Cook garlic and ginger for a short time over medium heat, stirring constantly. This will release their flavors without allowing them to burn. You can also consider adding them a bit later in the cooking process.

You need to understand that cooking is all about practice and experimentation. Don't be discouraged by challenges – they can be great learning opportunities!

Wholesome Sides and Snacks

In the hustle and bustle of modern life, maintaining a healthy and balanced diet often takes a backseat. However, the significance of incorporating wholesome sides and snacks into our daily eating habits cannot be overstated. These delectable treats not only tantalize our taste buds but also provide a plethora of health benefits that contribute to our overall well-being.

Nutritional Powerhouses:

Wholesome sides and snacks serve as nutritional powerhouses, delivering a wide array of essential nutrients that our bodies require to function optimally. From crunchy vegetables rich in vitamins and minerals to protein-packed nuts and seeds, these miniature meals provide a convenient way to ensure a well-rounded intake of nutrients. They are the secret behind keeping our bodies nourished and energized throughout the day.

Sustained Energy Release:

One of the primary advantages of incorporating wholesome sides and snacks into our daily routine is their ability to provide sustained energy release. Unlike sugary or processed snacks that result in quick energy spikes followed by crashes, wholesome options like whole grains, fruits, and lean proteins release energy gradually. This keeps us alert and focused, preventing the mid-afternoon energy slump that often plagues our productivity.

Weight Management and Portion Control:

For those striving to manage their weight, wholesome sides and snacks are invaluable allies. These nutrient-dense choices offer a sense of fullness, curbing unnecessary overeating during main meals. Moreover, they aid in portion control, preventing the temptation to indulge in calorie-laden, empty snacks. Thus, they play a crucial role in maintaining a healthy weight and preventing mindless munching.

Supporting Mental Health:

The connection between diet and mental health is becoming increasingly apparent. Wholesome sides and snacks that are rich in omega-3 fatty acids, antioxidants, and vitamins contribute to cognitive function and emotional well-being. Foods like nuts, seeds, and berries not only nourish our bodies but also support brain health, positively impacting our mood and overall mental state.

Versatility and Culinary Creativity:

Wholesome sides and snacks provide an exciting canvas for culinary creativity. With an assortment of ingredients at our disposal, we can craft a variety of delicious and visually appealing treats. From yogurt parfaits adorned with fresh fruits to vegetable platters paired with nutrient-rich dips, the possibilities are endless. This encourages us to experiment with flavors, textures, and combinations, making healthy eating an enjoyable endeavor.

Inclusivity and Special Diets:

For individuals with dietary restrictions or special preferences, wholesome sides and snacks offer a wide range of choices that accommodate various dietary needs. From gluten-free to vegan options, these treats ensure that everyone can indulge in flavorful and nourishing delights without compromising on taste or nutrition.

The role of wholesome sides and snacks extends far beyond their status as between-meal munchies. These miniature meals are the unsung heroes of our dietary choices, promoting optimal health, sustained energy, and mental well-being. By incorporating a variety of nutrient-rich options into our daily routine, we embark on a journey toward a healthier and more vibrant lifestyle. So, the next time you're tempted to reach for a sugary snack, consider the myriad benefits that wholesome sides and snacks bring to the table – quite literally!

<u>Baked Sweet Potato Fries</u>

Baked sweet potato fries are a popular and healthier alternative to traditional potato fries. They are made from sweet potatoes, which are rich in vitamins, minerals, and dietary fiber. To prepare them, sweet potatoes are cut into thin strips, seasoned with various spices like paprika, garlic powder, and cayenne pepper, and then baked in the oven until they become crispy.

One of the key benefits of baked sweet potato fries is that they are lower in calories and fat compared to deep-fried potato fries. They also have a lower glycemic index, which means they have a slower impact on blood sugar levels. This can be especially beneficial for those looking to manage their blood sugar.

The natural sweetness of sweet potatoes gives these fries a unique flavor profile that can be enhanced with different seasonings and dips. Common dipping options include yogurt-based sauces, aioli, ketchup, or even a sprinkle of cinnamon for a sweet twist.

When baking sweet potato fries, it's important to spread them out on the baking sheet to ensure even cooking and crispiness. Using parchment paper or lightly oiling the baking sheet can help prevent sticking. Also, remember that sweet potatoes have a higher moisture content than regular potatoes, so the fries might not become as crispy as traditional fries, but they still offer a delightful texture.

Overall, baked sweet potato fries are a nutritious and tasty alternative to regular fries, offering a satisfying side dish or snack option that is easy to customize to your taste preferences.

Baked Sweet Potato Fries Prep

Consider that the cooking times may vary based on the thickness of the fries and your oven, so keep an eye on them as they bake.

Let's delve into the process of preparing Baked Sweet Potato Fries:

1. Gather Ingredients:

- Sweet potatoes (2 large)

- Olive oil (2 tablespoons)

- Salt (1/2 teaspoon)

- Pepper (1/4 teaspoon)

- Optional seasonings (paprika, garlic powder, etc.)

2. Preheat the Oven:

- Preheat your oven to 425°F (220°C).

3. Wash and Peel:

- Wash and peel the sweet potatoes. Cut off the ends.

4. Cut into Fries:

- Cut the sweet potatoes into thin strips, resembling the shape of fries.

5. Soak in Water:

- Place the cut sweet potato strips in a bowl of cold water and let them soak for about 30 minutes. This helps remove excess starch and makes the fries crispier.

6. Dry and Season:

- Drain and pat dry the soaked sweet potato strips with paper towels.
- In a large bowl, toss the dry sweet potato strips with olive oil, salt, pepper, and any optional seasonings you like.

7. Arrange on Baking Sheet:

- Spread the seasoned sweet potato strips in a single layer on a baking sheet, making sure they don't overlap.

8. Bake:

- Place the baking sheet in the preheated oven and bake for about 20-25 minutes, or until the fries are golden and crispy, flipping them halfway through.

9. Serve:

- Once the sweet potato fries are baked to your desired crispiness, remove them from the oven.
- Let them cool slightly before serving.

10. Enjoy:

- Serve the baked sweet potato fries with your favorite dipping sauce, such as ketchup, aioli, or yogurt-based sauces.

<u>Baked Sweet Potato Fries Prep Challenges and Solutions</u>

Here are some potential problems that might arise during the preparation of Baked Sweet Potato Fries and their corresponding solutions:

<u>Problem 1: Soggy Fries</u>

- Soaking the sweet potato strips for too long or not drying them properly can result in soggy fries.

- **Solution:** Ensure you only soak the sweet potato strips for about 30 minutes and pat them dry thoroughly with paper towels before seasoning and baking.

<u>Problem 2: Uneven Cooking</u>

- If the sweet potato strips are not cut to a consistent size, they might cook unevenly.

- Solution: Aim for uniform cuts to ensure even cooking. You can use a mandoline slicer or knife to achieve consistent thickness.

Problem 3: Overcrowding on the Baking Sheet

- If the sweet potato strips are crowded on the baking sheet, they may not crisp up properly.

- Solution: Spread the sweet potato strips in a single layer on the baking sheet, leaving some space between each strip. You may need to use multiple baking sheets if necessary.

Problem 4: Burning

- Baking at too high a temperature or not flipping the fries halfway through can result in burning.

- **Solution:** Follow the recommended baking temperature and duration. Flip the fries halfway through to ensure even browning and prevent burning.

Problem 5: Lack of Seasoning

- For bland fries, not using enough seasoning can be an issue.

- **Solution:** Toss the sweet potato strips with an appropriate amount of olive oil, salt, pepper, and any optional seasonings you prefer, ensuring they are evenly coated.

Problem 6: Sticking to the Baking Sheet

- If the sweet potato strips stick to the baking sheet, they can break apart when trying to remove them.

- **Solution:** Use parchment paper or a silicone baking mat on the baking sheet to prevent sticking. You can also lightly grease the baking sheet.

143

Problem 7: Undercooked Fries

- Undercooking the fries can result in a chewy texture.

- **Solution:** Make sure to bake the sweet potato fries until they are golden and crispy. You can use a fork to test their doneness – they should be tender on the inside and crisp on the outside.

Problem 8: Seasoning Clumping

- If the seasoning clumps together instead of distributing evenly, the flavor won't be consistent.

- **Solution:** Mix the seasoning well with the sweet potato strips in a large bowl to ensure an even distribution of flavor.

By being mindful of these potential problems and implementing the suggested solutions, you can increase your chances of successfully preparing delicious Baked Sweet Potato Fries.

Cucumber and Carrot Sticks with Hummus

When it comes to healthy and delicious snacks, cucumber and carrot sticks with hummus are a winning combination that satisfies both the palate and the body. This wholesome snack is not only visually appealing but also packed with nutrients that contribute to overall well-being.

The star of this ensemble, cucumber, brings a refreshing crunch and a high water content that helps to keep you hydrated. Its mild flavor provides a neutral base that pairs perfectly with the robust taste of hummus. Carrot sticks, on the other hand, bring a touch of natural sweetness and a vibrant orange hue that appeals to both children and adults alike.

The real hero of this snack, though, is the hummus. Made from a blend of chickpeas, tahini, olive oil, lemon juice, and various seasonings, hummus not only enhances the flavor of the vegetables but also offers a plethora of health benefits. Chickpeas are a rich source of plant-based protein and fiber, which help to keep you full and provide sustained energy. The healthy fats from olive oil and tahini contribute to a feeling of satiety and support heart health.

This snack isn't just about taste – it's a nutritional powerhouse. The combination of vegetables and hummus provides a balance of carbohydrates, proteins, and fats, making it an ideal option for a midday pick-me-up or a pre-workout snack. Additionally, the fiber content aids in digestion and supports gut health.

Preparing cucumber and carrot sticks with hummus is a simple endeavor that can be enjoyed by anyone. Wash and cut the vegetables into easy-to-hold sticks, and arrange them neatly on a plate alongside a bowl of hummus. The colorful arrangement is not only inviting but also encourages mindful eating, making each bite a moment of delight and nourishment.

Cucumber and carrot sticks with hummus are a delightful snack that combines the crispness of vegetables with the creamy goodness of hummus. This pairing offers a satisfying blend of flavors and textures while delivering a host of nutrients that contribute to a healthier lifestyle. So, the next time you're looking for a quick, tasty, and nutritious snack, reach for a plate of cucumber and carrot sticks with hummus – your taste buds and body will thank you.

Cucumber and Carrot Sticks with Hummus prep

1. Gather Ingredients:

- 1 cucumber

- 2 carrots

- 1 cup hummus

- Salt and pepper (optional)

2. Wash and Peel:

- Wash the cucumber and carrots thoroughly.

- Peel the carrots and trim the ends of the cucumber.

3. Cut Vegetables:

- Cut the cucumber and carrots into long, thin sticks.

- Aim for uniform sizes for a visually appealing presentation.

4. Prepare Hummus:

- If you're making hummus from scratch, blend:

- 1 can (15 oz) chickpeas (drained and rinsed)

- 1/4 cup tahini

- 3 tablespoons lemon juice

- 2 cloves garlic

- 2 tablespoons olive oil

- Salt and cumin to taste

- Water (as needed for desired consistency)

5. Season Hummus (Optional):

- Add salt, pepper, and other seasonings to taste.

- Adjust consistency by adding a little water if necessary.

6. Arrange on a Plate:

- Place the cucumber and carrot sticks on a serving plate.

7. Serve with Hummus:

- Put the bowl of hummus in the center of the plate.

- Optionally, drizzle a bit of olive oil and sprinkle paprika on the hummus.

8. Enjoy:

- Dip the cucumber and carrot sticks into the hummus and enjoy your healthy snack!

Be aware that the quantities and steps are just an example. Adjustments can be made based on the number of servings you need and your personal preferences.

Cucumber and Carrot Sticks with Hummus Prep Challenges and Solutions

These are the Problems and Solutions encountered for Cucumber and Carrot Sticks with Hummus Snacking:

Problems:

1. **Availability:** Finding fresh and high-quality cucumbers and carrots year-round might be a challenge, impacting the taste and nutritional value of the snack.

 - **Solution:** Consider shopping at local farmer's markets or opting for frozen vegetables during off-seasons to ensure freshness and taste.

2. **Dipping Portion Control:** It's easy to unconsciously overindulge in hummus, which could lead to excessive calorie intake.

- **Solution:** Pre-portion the hummus into small containers or use a kitchen scale to measure out a reasonable serving size.

3. **Nutritional Balance:** While hummus provides healthy fats and protein, it's still important to ensure a well-rounded snack with a balanced nutritional profile.

- **Solution:** Incorporate other dips like Greek yogurt-based tzatziki or add a side of nuts for extra protein and healthy fats.

4. **Travel and On-the-Go:** Carrying fresh vegetables and hummus might not be convenient when you're away from home.

- **Solution:** Prep and pack the snack in advance using airtight containers or consider purchasing pre-packaged single-serving hummus cups.

5. Boredom and Variety: Eating the same snack repeatedly could lead to taste fatigue.

- **Solution:** Experiment with different veggie options (bell peppers, celery, etc.) and explore various hummus flavors (roasted red pepper, garlic, etc.) to keep the snack interesting.

6. Sustainability: Purchasing pre-packaged hummus and individually wrapped vegetables can generate excess waste.

- **Solution:** Make your hummus at home using bulk chickpeas and reusable containers for both hummus and veggies.

7. Allergies and Dietary Restrictions: Some individuals might be allergic to ingredients in hummus, like sesame (found in tahini).

- **Solution:** Explore alternative dips like guacamole or nut-based spreads for those with allergies, and always check ingredient labels.

8. Social Situations: In group settings, double-dipping or sharing communal dips might lead to hygiene concerns.

- Solution: Opt for individually portioned snacks or provide serving utensils to maintain hygiene and courtesy.

9. Time and Preparation: Washing, peeling, and cutting vegetables can be time-consuming.

- **Solution:** Dedicate time for meal prep during the week to wash, peel, and cut veggies in advance, making snack assembly quick and hassle-free.

10. Texture and Palate Preferences: Some people might not enjoy the texture or taste of raw vegetables and hummus.

- **Solution:** Modify the snack to suit personal preferences by lightly roasting the vegetables or trying a different dip altogether.

Addressing these problems and implementing the solutions can make the experience of enjoying cucumber and carrot sticks with hummus both convenient and delightful while ensuring you're making the most of its nutritional benefits.

Black Bean Tacos with Mango Salsa Probs and Solutions

Some potential problems might arise while preparing "Black Bean Tacos with Mango Salsa," along with their corresponding solutions:

Problem 1: Overly salty salsa

- If the mango salsa turns out too salty:

Solution: Taste and adjust the seasoning. You can add more diced mango or a squeeze of lime juice to balance out the saltiness.

Problem 2: Dry or flavorless beans

- If the black bean mixture is too dry or lacks flavor:

Solution: Add a splash of vegetable broth or water to the black bean mixture to add moisture and enhance the flavor. You can also adjust the seasoning by adding more cumin and chili powder.

Problem 3: Tortillas are difficult to work with

- If the corn tortillas are cracking or breaking when you try to fold them:

Solution: Heat the tortillas properly until they are soft and pliable. You can do this by briefly warming them in a skillet or over an open flame. Additionally, consider using two tortillas per taco to make them more sturdy.

Problem 4: Mango salsa is too tangy

- If the mango salsa is too tangy from the lime juice:

Solution: Balance out the tanginess by adding a bit more diced mango or a pinch of sugar to the salsa.

Problem 5: Tacos are falling apart

- If the tacos are falling apart when you try to eat them:

Solution: Make sure to not overfill the tacos. Start with a spoonful of the black bean mixture and then layer the mango salsa and other toppings. If the tortillas are too delicate, you can also double them up to make them sturdier.

Problem 6: Tacos are too bland

- If the overall flavor of the tacos is too bland:

Solution: Be sure to season each component well. Add more cumin, chili powder, or salt as needed. You can also consider adding some extra toppings like sliced jalapeños or a drizzle of hot sauce for added flavor.

<u>Mushroom and Spinach Stir-Fry</u>

Mushroom and spinach stir-fry is a delightful and nutritious dish that brings together the earthy flavors of mushrooms and the vibrant freshness of spinach. This simple yet flavorful recipe is a perfect choice for those seeking a quick and healthy meal option.

To begin, gather the ingredients: fresh mushrooms (such as button or cremini), fresh spinach leaves, garlic, onions, soy sauce, and your choice of cooking oil. Start by cleaning and slicing the mushrooms into thin pieces. Next, wash and pat dry the spinach leaves, removing any tough stems.

In a heated pan, add a dash of cooking oil and sauté finely chopped garlic and onions until they turn translucent. Then, add the sliced mushrooms and let them cook until they release their moisture and start to brown. The aroma that fills the kitchen at this stage is truly enticing.

Once the mushrooms are nicely cooked, it's time to add the fresh spinach leaves. The spinach will wilt quickly, so it's essential to keep stirring gently. As the leaves begin to wilt, drizzle in some soy sauce for flavor and a touch of saltiness.

In just a few minutes, the spinach will be perfectly cooked, retaining its vibrant green color. The mushrooms and spinach will have absorbed the flavors of the garlic, onions, and soy sauce, creating a harmonious blend of tastes.

This mushroom and spinach stir-fry can be served as a standalone dish or paired with steamed rice, quinoa, or noodles. For those who enjoy a bit of heat, a sprinkle of red pepper flakes or a dash of hot sauce can add an exciting kick.

Not only does this dish tantalize your taste buds, but it's also a nutritional powerhouse. Spinach is rich in vitamins and minerals, while mushrooms offer a good dose of protein and immune-boosting properties.

The mushroom and spinach stir-fry is a testament to the beauty of simplicity in cooking. With just a handful of ingredients and minimal effort, you can create a wholesome and flavorful meal that satisfies both the palate and the body. So, whether you're a seasoned chef or a beginner in the kitchen, this dish is a must-try for its ease, taste, and nutritional value.

Mushroom and Spinach Stir-Fry

An itemized process for preparing Mushroom and Spinach Stir-Fry is as follows:

Ingredients:

- 250g mushrooms, sliced

- 200g spinach, washed and chopped

- 1 tablespoon olive oil

- 2 cloves garlic, minced

- 1 teaspoon ginger, minced

- 1 tablespoon soy sauce

- 1/2 teaspoon sesame oil

- Salt and pepper to taste

- Optional: red pepper flakes for some heat

Instructions:

1. Heat the olive oil in a large pan over medium-high heat.

2. Add the minced garlic and ginger. Sauté for about 30 seconds until fragrant.

3. Add the sliced mushrooms and cook for 3-4 minutes until they start to soften and release their moisture.

4. Stir in the chopped spinach and cook for an additional 2-3 minutes until wilted.

5. Drizzle in the soy sauce and sesame oil, and give everything a good stir to combine.

6. Season with salt, pepper, and red pepper flakes if using. Adjust seasoning to taste.

7. Continue to cook for another 1-2 minutes, allowing the flavors to meld together.

8. Remove from heat and serve the Mushroom and Spinach Stir-fry immediately as a side dish or overcooked rice or noodles.

Mushroom and Spinach Stir-Fry Challenges and Solutions

These are challenges that you might encounter while preparing Mushroom and Spinach Stir-Fry, along with possible solutions as follows:

Challenges:

1. Mushroom Moisture: Mushrooms release a lot of moisture when cooked, which can lead to a soggy stir-fry.

 Solution: To prevent this, make sure the pan is hot before adding the mushrooms. Cook them in batches if necessary, allowing space between slices for moisture to evaporate. High heat will help evaporate excess moisture.

2. Overcooking Spinach: Spinach can quickly go from fresh to wilted and overcooked.

Solution: Add spinach towards the end of cooking to prevent overcooking. Stir it in for just a couple of minutes until it wilts, and then remove from heat promptly.

3. Flavor Balance: Achieving the right balance of flavors, especially between the soy sauce and sesame oil, can be tricky.

Solution: Start with a small amount of soy sauce and sesame oil, and taste as you go. You can always add more, but you can't take it away. Remember that you can adjust the seasoning at the end.

4. Texture Concerns: Overcooking mushrooms can result in a rubbery texture, and if spinach is overcooked, it can become mushy.

Solution: Keep a close eye on the cooking time and use high heat for mushrooms to achieve a nice sear. Aim for vibrant green spinach, not a mushy texture.

5. Garlic and Ginger Burning: Minced garlic and ginger can burn quickly, resulting in a bitter taste.

Solution: Cook garlic and ginger for a short time over medium heat, stirring constantly. This will release their flavors without allowing them to burn. You can also consider adding them a bit later in the cooking process.

You need to understand that cooking is all about practice and experimentation. Don't be discouraged by challenges – they can be great learning opportunities!

<u>Wholesome Sides and Snacks</u>

In the hustle and bustle of modern life, maintaining a healthy and balanced diet often takes a backseat. However, the significance of incorporating wholesome sides and snacks into our daily eating habits cannot be overstated. These delectable treats not only tantalize our taste buds but also provide a plethora of health benefits that contribute to our overall well-being.

<u>Nutritional Powerhouses:</u>

Wholesome sides and snacks serve as nutritional powerhouses, delivering a wide array of essential nutrients that our bodies require to function optimally. From crunchy vegetables rich in vitamins and minerals to protein-packed nuts and seeds, these miniature meals provide a convenient way to ensure a well-rounded intake of nutrients. They are the secret behind keeping our bodies nourished and energized throughout the day.

Sustained Energy Release:

One of the primary advantages of incorporating wholesome sides and snacks into our daily routine is their ability to provide sustained energy release. Unlike sugary or processed snacks that result in quick energy spikes followed by crashes, wholesome options like whole grains, fruits, and lean proteins release energy gradually. This keeps us alert and focused, preventing the mid-afternoon energy slump that often plagues our productivity.

Weight Management and Portion Control:

For those striving to manage their weight, wholesome sides and snacks are invaluable allies. These nutrient-dense choices offer a sense of fullness, curbing unnecessary overeating during main meals. Moreover, they aid in portion control, preventing the temptation to indulge in calorie-laden, empty snacks. Thus, they play a crucial role in maintaining a healthy weight and preventing mindless munching.

Supporting Mental Health:

The connection between diet and mental health is becoming increasingly apparent. Wholesome sides and snacks that are rich in omega-3 fatty acids, antioxidants, and vitamins contribute to cognitive function and emotional well-being. Foods like nuts, seeds, and berries not only nourish our bodies but also support brain health, positively impacting our mood and overall mental state.

Versatility and Culinary Creativity:

Wholesome sides and snacks provide an exciting canvas for culinary creativity. With an assortment of ingredients at our disposal, we can craft a variety of delicious and visually appealing treats. From yogurt parfaits adorned with fresh fruits to vegetable platters paired with nutrient-rich dips, the possibilities are endless. This encourages us to experiment with flavors, textures, and combinations, making healthy eating an enjoyable endeavor.

<u>Inclusivity and Special Diets:</u>

For individuals with dietary restrictions or special preferences, wholesome sides and snacks offer a wide range of choices that accommodate various dietary needs. From gluten-free to vegan options, these treats ensure that everyone can indulge in flavorful and nourishing delights without compromising on taste or nutrition.

The role of wholesome sides and snacks extends far beyond their status as between-meal munchies. These miniature meals are the unsung heroes of our dietary choices, promoting optimal health, sustained energy, and mental well-being. By incorporating a variety of nutrient-rich options into our daily routine, we embark on a journey toward a healthier and more vibrant lifestyle. So, the next time you're tempted to reach for a sugary snack, consider the myriad benefits that wholesome sides and snacks bring to the table – quite literally!

Baked Sweet Potato Fries

Baked sweet potato fries are a popular and healthier alternative to traditional potato fries. They are made from sweet potatoes, which are rich in vitamins, minerals, and dietary fiber. To prepare them, sweet potatoes are cut into thin strips, seasoned with various spices like paprika, garlic powder, and cayenne pepper, and then baked in the oven until they become crispy.

One of the key benefits of baked sweet potato fries is that they are lower in calories and fat compared to deep-fried potato fries. They also have a lower glycemic index, which means they have a slower impact on blood sugar levels. This can be especially beneficial for those looking to manage their blood sugar.

The natural sweetness of sweet potatoes gives these fries a unique flavor profile that can be enhanced with different seasonings and dips. Common dipping options include yogurt-based sauces, aioli, ketchup, or even a sprinkle of cinnamon for a sweet twist.

When baking sweet potato fries, it's important to spread them out on the baking sheet to ensure even cooking and crispiness. Using parchment paper or lightly oiling the baking sheet can help prevent sticking. Also, remember that sweet potatoes have a higher moisture content than regular potatoes, so the fries might not become as crispy as traditional fries, but they still offer a delightful texture.

Overall, baked sweet potato fries are a nutritious and tasty alternative to regular fries, offering a satisfying side dish or snack option that is easy to customize to your taste preferences.

Baked Sweet Potato Fries Prep

Consider that the cooking times may vary based on the thickness of the fries and your oven, so keep an eye on them as they bake.

Let's delve into the process of preparing Baked Sweet Potato Fries:

1. Gather Ingredients:

- Sweet potatoes (2 large)

- Olive oil (2 tablespoons)

- Salt (1/2 teaspoon)

- Pepper (1/4 teaspoon)

- Optional seasonings (paprika, garlic powder, etc.)

2. Preheat the Oven:

- Preheat your oven to 425°F (220°C).

3. Wash and Peel:

- Wash and peel the sweet potatoes. Cut off the ends.

4. Cut into Fries:

- Cut the sweet potatoes into thin strips, resembling the shape of fries.

5. Soak in Water:

- Place the cut sweet potato strips in a bowl of cold water and let them soak for about 30 minutes. This helps remove excess starch and makes the fries crispier.

6. Dry and Season:

- Drain and pat dry the soaked sweet potato strips with paper towels.
- In a large bowl, toss the dry sweet potato strips with olive oil, salt, pepper, and any optional seasonings you like.

7. Arrange on Baking Sheet:

- Spread the seasoned sweet potato strips in a single layer on a baking sheet, making sure they don't overlap.

8. Bake:

- Place the baking sheet in the preheated oven and bake for about 20-25 minutes, or until the fries are golden and crispy, flipping them halfway through.

9. Serve:

- Once the sweet potato fries are baked to your desired crispiness, remove them from the oven.
- Let them cool slightly before serving.

10. Enjoy:

- Serve the baked sweet potato fries with your favorite dipping sauce, such as ketchup, aioli, or yogurt-based sauces.

Baked Sweet Potato Fries Prep Challenges and Solutions

Sure, here are some potential problems that might arise during the preparation of Baked Sweet Potato Fries and their corresponding solutions:

Problem 1: Soggy Fries

- Soaking the sweet potato strips for too long or not drying them properly can result in soggy fries.

- **Solution:** Ensure you only soak the sweet potato strips for about 30 minutes and pat them dry thoroughly with paper towels before seasoning and baking.

Problem 2: Uneven Cooking

- If the sweet potato strips are not cut to a consistent size, they might cook unevenly.

- **Solution:** Aim for uniform cuts to ensure even cooking. You can use a mandoline slicer or knife to achieve consistent thickness.

Problem 3: Overcrowding on the Baking Sheet

- If the sweet potato strips are crowded on the baking sheet, they may not crisp up properly.

- **Solution:** Spread the sweet potato strips in a single layer on the baking sheet, leaving some space between each strip. You may need to use multiple baking sheets if necessary.

Problem 4: Burning

- Baking at too high a temperature or not flipping the fries halfway through can result in burning.

- **Solution:** Follow the recommended baking temperature and duration. Flip the fries halfway through to ensure even browning and prevent burning.

Problem 5: Lack of Seasoning

- For bland fries, not using enough seasoning can be an issue.

- **Solution:** Toss the sweet potato strips with an appropriate amount of olive oil, salt, pepper, and any optional seasonings you prefer, ensuring they are evenly coated.

Problem 6: Sticking to the Baking Sheet

- If the sweet potato strips stick to the baking sheet, they can break apart when trying to remove them.

- **Solution:** Use parchment paper or a silicone baking mat on the baking sheet to prevent sticking. You can also lightly grease the baking sheet.

Problem 7: Undercooked Fries

- Undercooking the fries can result in a chewy texture.

- **Solution:** Make sure to bake the sweet potato fries until they are golden and crispy. You can use a fork to test their doneness – they should be tender on the inside and crisp on the outside.

Problem 8: Seasoning Clumping

- If the seasoning clumps together instead of distributing evenly, the flavor won't be consistent.
- **Solution:** Mix the seasoning well with the sweet potato strips in a large bowl to ensure an even distribution of flavor.

By being mindful of these potential problems and implementing the suggested solutions, you can increase your chances of successfully preparing delicious Baked Sweet Potato Fries.

Roasted Brussels Sprouts

Brussels sprouts, with their delightful blend of flavors and textures, have become a staple on many dining tables, elevating the humble vegetable to gourmet status. These miniature cabbage-like orbs have transformed, turning from a potentially dreaded side dish to a savory sensation that tantalizes taste buds.

The process of roasting works its magic on Brussels sprouts, infusing them with a nutty, caramelized essence that adds depth to their natural earthiness. Preparing them is a straightforward task: After washing and trimming, the sprouts are tossed in olive oil, seasoned with a pinch of salt and pepper, and then laid out on a baking sheet. The high heat of the oven coaxes out their natural sugars, resulting in a crispy exterior and a tender interior.

The beauty of roasted Brussels sprouts lies in their versatility. They act as a blank canvas, ready to be adorned with an array of complementary flavors. A drizzle of balsamic glaze adds a touch of sweetness, while a sprinkle of grated Parmesan cheese introduces a hint of umami. The addition of toasted almonds or crumbled bacon contributes a satisfying crunch, creating a medley of textures that dance on the palate.

Nutritionally, Brussels sprouts are a powerhouse, packed with vitamins, fiber, and antioxidants. Roasting retains much of its nutritional value, making it not only delicious but also a health-conscious choice. Their ability to absorb flavors makes them an ideal ingredient to experiment with various seasonings, turning an ordinary side dish into a culinary adventure.

In conclusion, the rise of roasted Brussels sprouts in the culinary world is a testament to the transformative power of cooking techniques. From their initial reputation as a vegetable to be avoided, they have emerged as a delectable delight that showcases the artistry of cooking. Whether enjoyed as a simple side dish or dressed up with a medley of flavors, roasted Brussels sprouts are a testament to the fact that even the most humble ingredients can be elevated to culinary greatness.

Roasted Brussels Sprouts Prep

Ingredients:

- 1 pound (450g) Brussels sprouts

- 2 tablespoons olive oil

- 1/2 teaspoon salt

- 1/4 teaspoon black pepper

- Optional: 2 tablespoons balsamic glaze, 1/4 cup grated Parmesan cheese, 1/4 cup toasted almonds or crumbled bacon

Instructions:

1. **Preheat the Oven:** Preheat your oven to 400°F (200°C).

2. **Prepare the Brussels Sprouts:** Wash the Brussels sprouts thoroughly and trim the ends. If they are large, you can cut them in half for more even cooking.

3. Toss with Olive Oil: In a mixing bowl, toss the Brussels sprouts with 2 tablespoons of olive oil. Make sure they are evenly coated.

4. Season: Sprinkle 1/2 teaspoon of salt and 1/4 teaspoon of black pepper over the Brussels sprouts. Toss again to distribute the seasoning.

5. Arrange on Baking Sheet: Line a baking sheet with parchment paper or lightly grease it. Spread the seasoned Brussels sprouts evenly on the baking sheet in a single layer.

6. Roast: Place the baking sheet in the preheated oven and roast the Brussels sprouts for about 20-25 minutes, or until they are golden brown and crispy on the edges. You can gently toss them halfway through the cooking time for even roasting.

7. Optional Flavors: If desired, you can take the roasted Brussels sprouts out of the oven a few minutes before they are done and drizzle them with balsamic glaze. You can also sprinkle grated Parmesan cheese or toasted almonds/crumbled bacon over the top for added flavor and texture.

8. Serve: Once roasted to your liking, remove the Brussels sprouts from the oven. Transfer them to a serving dish and enjoy them as a delightful side dish or even as a standalone snack.

Understand that the cooking times may vary based on the size of the Brussels sprouts and your oven, so keep an eye on them as they roast to ensure they don't overcook.

Problems and Solutions When Roasting Brussels Sprouts

Problem 1: Uneven Roasting

- **Issue:** Brussels sprouts are roasting unevenly, with some parts getting too brown while others remain undercooked.

- **Solution:** Make sure the Brussels sprouts are cut to a similar size to ensure even cooking. Consider tossing them halfway through the roasting time to promote even browning on all sides.

Problem 2: Dry Brussels Sprouts

- **Issue:** The roasted Brussels sprouts turned out dry and lacking in flavor.

- **Solution:** Increase the amount of olive oil used for coating before roasting. This will help the sprouts retain moisture and enhance their flavor. You can also add more seasoning or experiment with different seasonings for more flavor.

Problem 3: Overly Bitter Brussels Sprouts

- **Issue:** The roasted Brussels sprouts have a bitter taste.

- **Solution:** Bitterness can be reduced by choosing smaller and fresher Brussels sprouts. You can also blanch them briefly in boiling water before roasting them to mellow out the bitterness.

Problem 4: Brussels Sprouts are Soggy

- **Issue:** The roasted Brussels sprouts are turning out soggy instead of crispy.

- **Solution:** Ensure that the Brussels sprouts are well-dried before tossing them with olive oil. Excess moisture can hinder crisping. Additionally, avoid overcrowding the baking sheet to allow proper air circulation, which is crucial for achieving crispiness.

Problem 5: Lack of Flavor Variation

- **Issue:** The roasted Brussels sprouts taste one-dimensional and lack variety.

- **Solution:** Experiment with different flavor additions to enhance the taste. Try drizzling with balsamic glaze, adding grated Parmesan cheese, or incorporating toasted nuts or crumbled bacon for different textures and flavors.

Problem 6: Brussels Sprouts Burn Quickly

- **Issue:** The Brussels sprouts are burning or getting too dark too quickly.

- **Solution:** Lower the oven temperature slightly or reduce the roasting time. Keep an eye on them as they roast to prevent overcooking. You can also cover the

Brussels sprouts loosely with aluminum foil during roasting to slow down browning if needed.

Problem 7: Brussels Sprouts are Undercooked

- **Issue:** The roasted Brussels sprouts are still too firm and undercooked.

- **Solution:** Increase the roasting time by 5-10 minutes and check for doneness. If they are still too firm, continue roasting in 5-minute increments until they are tender when pierced with a fork.

Problem 8: Lack of Crispy Texture

- **Issue:** The Brussels sprouts are not achieving the desired crispy texture.

- **Solution:** Ensure that the oven is preheated to the correct temperature. You can also try increasing the roasting time slightly or broiling them for a minute or two at the end of cooking to achieve the desired crispiness.

Easy One-Pot Meals: Simplicity and Flavor in a Single Pot

In today's fast-paced world, the demand for convenient yet delicious meals is on the rise. Enter the realm of one-pot meals, a culinary trend that has captured the hearts and taste buds of many. With their straightforward preparation and minimal clean-up, one-pot meals offer a practical solution for busy individuals seeking a satisfying home-cooked meal.

One of the key advantages of one-pot meals is their versatility. Whether you're a meat lover, a vegetarian, or someone with specific dietary restrictions, there's a one-pot recipe to suit your taste. Imagine the aroma of a hearty chicken and vegetable stew simmering on the stove or the comfort of a creamy risotto infused with herbs and Parmesan cheese.

Furthermore, the convenience factor cannot be overstated. With just a single pot to clean, the post-meal cleanup becomes a breeze. This is a boon for busy individuals who wish to enjoy a homemade meal without spending hours in the kitchen or facing a mountain of dirty dishes afterward.

For those with a penchant for culinary creativity, one-pot meals can be a canvas for experimentation. Add spices, herbs, and seasonings to elevate the flavor profile. Swap ingredients to cater to personal preferences or use up what's available in the pantry. The flexibility of one-pot cooking allows for both novice and experienced cooks to explore and innovate.

Incorporating one-pot meals into your routine can also contribute to reduced food waste. Leftover vegetables, meats, or grains can find new life in a colorful and flavorful medley, minimizing the need to discard unused portions.

Easy one-pot meals are a testament to the fusion of convenience and culinary delight. With their straightforward preparation, versatile options, and efficient cleanup, they cater to the demands of modern life while ensuring that the joy of a home-cooked meal remains intact. So, whether you're a busy professional, a student, or anyone looking for a quick yet wholesome meal, one-pot cooking might just be your ticket to a satisfying dining experience.

<u>Easy One-Pot Meals Prep</u>

Certainly, here's an itemized process for preparing a simple one-pot chicken and vegetable stir-fry for 2 servings:

<u>Ingredients:</u>

- 1 boneless chicken breast, thinly sliced

- 1 cup broccoli florets

- 1 medium carrot, julienned

- 1 red bell pepper, thinly sliced

- 1 cup cooked rice

- 2 tablespoons soy sauce

- 1 tablespoon vegetable oil

- 1 teaspoon minced garlic

- 1 teaspoon minced ginger

- Salt and pepper to taste

- Chopped green onions for garnish

Instructions:

1. Heat the Oil: Place a large skillet or wok over medium-high heat. Add the vegetable oil and let it heat up.

2. Sauté the Aromatics: Add the minced garlic and ginger to the hot oil. Sauté for about 30 seconds until fragrant.

3. Cook the Chicken: Add the sliced chicken to the skillet. Cook, stirring occasionally, until the chicken is cooked through and no longer pink, about 5-7 minutes.

4. Add the Vegetables: Toss in the julienned carrot, broccoli florets, and red bell pepper. Stir-fry for another 3-4 minutes until the vegetables are slightly tender but still crisp.

5. Season: Pour in the soy sauce and give everything a good mix. Season with salt and pepper according to your taste.

6. Incorporate Rice: Push the chicken and vegetables to the side of the skillet, creating a space in the center. Add the cooked rice to the center of the skillet. Allow it to heat up for a minute or two.

7. Combine and Stir-Fry: Gradually combine the rice with the chicken and vegetables, mixing everything. Stir-fry for an additional 2-3 minutes to let the flavors meld.

8. Taste and Adjust: Taste the stir-fry and adjust the seasoning if necessary. You can add a bit more soy sauce or salt if desired.

9. Serve: Once everything is heated through and well combined, remove the skillet from heat. Divide the stir-fry into two serving plates.

10. Garnish: Sprinkle chopped green onions over the stir-fry for a fresh and vibrant finish.

11. Enjoy: Your delicious one-pot chicken and vegetable stir-fry is now ready to be enjoyed!

The beauty of one-pot meals is that you can modify the ingredients and quantities to suit your preferences.

Easy One-Pot Meals Pre-Problems and Solutions

Here's is an itemized list of common problems that can arise when preparing one-pot meals, along with corresponding solutions:

Problem: Ingredients are unevenly cooked.

- **Solution:** Ensure that you cut ingredients to similar sizes to promote even cooking. Start cooking the harder vegetables and proteins first before adding quicker-cooking items.

Problem: The dish lacks flavor or seasoning.

- **Solution:** Use a variety of spices, herbs, and seasonings to enhance the flavor. Taste and adjust as you go, adding salt, pepper, and sauces gradually to achieve the desired taste.

Problem: Rice or pasta becomes mushy.

- **Solution:** Follow recommended cooking times for rice and pasta. Consider slightly undercooking them since they'll continue to cook when combined with other ingredients.

Problem: Ingredients stick to the pot.

- **Solution:** Make sure to heat the pot or pan before adding oil. Keep the heat at an appropriate level and use enough oil to prevent sticking. Stir frequently to avoid burning.

Problem: The dish turns out too dry or too watery.

- **Solution:** Adjust the amount of liquid you add based on the ingredients and recipe. If it's too dry, add a bit of broth, water, or sauce. If it's too watery, let it simmer uncovered to reduce the liquid.

Problem: Overcooking ingredients.

- **Solution:** Pay attention to cooking times and avoid overcooking delicate ingredients like leafy greens or seafood. Add more delicate ingredients later in the cooking process.

Problem: Ingredients become mushy from prolonged cooking.

- **Solution:** Add ingredients that cook quickly towards the end. This helps maintain texture and prevents ingredients from becoming overly soft.

Problem: Ingredients lose their vibrant color.

- **Solution:** Briefly blanch or steam vegetables before adding them to the dish. Alternatively, add colorful ingredients towards the end of cooking to preserve their vibrancy.

Problem: The dish lacks variety.

- **Solution:** Mix and match ingredients based on your preferences and what you have on hand. Experiment with different proteins, vegetables, and grains to keep things interesting.

Problem: Inconsistent heat distribution.

- **Solution:** Stir the contents of the pot occasionally to distribute heat evenly. If using a stovetop, consider using a heavy-bottomed pot or pan to help distribute heat more effectively.

Problem: The dish is too salty or too bland.

- **Solution:** Taste as you go and adjust the seasoning accordingly. If a dish is too salty, balance it with a bit of acidity (e.g., lemon juice). If it's too bland, add more herbs and spices.

Problem: Cooking time is longer than expected.

- **Solution:** Plan and make sure you allocate enough time for the meal. Prepare ingredients in advance to streamline the cooking process.

One-Pot Lentil Curry

Lentils, with their incredible versatility and rich nutritional profile, have been a staple in various cuisines for centuries. Among the many ways to enjoy lentils, the one-pot lentil curry stands out as a hearty and satisfying dish that combines convenience, taste, and health benefits in a single pot.

A one-pot lentil curry is a culinary masterpiece that marries the earthy goodness of lentils with a harmonious blend of spices and aromatics.

The star of the dish, the lentils, takes center stage as they soak up the flavors of the spices and aromatics. Red, green, brown, or black lentils, each bring their unique texture and taste to the dish. As the lentils simmer and soften, they create a velvety base that becomes the canvas for the curry's robust character.

To elevate the nutritional quotient of the dish, many versions of one-pot lentil curry include an assortment of vegetables. Bell peppers, carrots, tomatoes, and spinach add vibrant colors and an array of vitamins and minerals. This not only enhances the dish's visual appeal but also provides a balanced and wholesome meal.

One of the most alluring aspects of the one-pot lentil curry is its simplicity. As the name suggests, all the magic happens in a single pot, making it an ideal choice for busy days or when you want to minimize the post-cooking cleanup. This simplicity, however, doesn't compromise the dish's complexity of flavors. The slow-cooking process allows the ingredients to meld and develop their tastes, resulting in a dish that's deeply satisfying with every spoonful.

Whether enjoyed with steamed rice, fluffy naan, or crusty bread, the one-pot lentil curry offers a delightful experience for the taste buds. Its warmth and comfort make it a favorite during cooler months, while its wholesome ingredients ensure that it remains a nutritious choice year-round.

The one-pot lentil curry is a testament to the culinary art of combining simple ingredients to create a dish that's greater than the sum of its parts. With its aromatic spices, nourishing lentils, and vibrant vegetables, this curry brings together flavor, convenience, and healthfulness in every bite. So, whether you're a seasoned cook or a novice in the kitchen, embark on the journey of crafting your one-pot lentil curry and savor the wonders it brings to your plate.

One-pot lentil curry Prep

Ingredients:

- 1 cup dried lentils (red, green, brown, or black)

- 1 onion, finely chopped

- 3 cloves of garlic, minced

- 1-inch piece of ginger, minced

- 2 tomatoes, chopped

- 1 cup mixed vegetables (bell peppers, carrots, spinach, etc.), chopped

- 2 tablespoons oil

- 1 teaspoon cumin seeds

- 1 teaspoon ground cumin

- 1 teaspoon ground coriander

- 1/2 teaspoon turmeric powder

- 1/2 teaspoon red chili powder (adjust to taste)

- 1/2 teaspoon garam masala

- Salt to taste

- 3 cups water or vegetable broth

- Fresh cilantro leaves for garnish.

Instructions:

1. Rinse the Lentils: Start by rinsing the lentils under cold water until the water runs clear. This helps remove any dirt or debris.

2. Sauté Aromatics: Heat the oil in a large pot over medium heat. Add the cumin seeds and let them sizzle for a few seconds. Then, add the chopped onions, minced garlic, and minced ginger. Sauté until the onions are translucent and aromatic.

3. Add Spices: Stir in the ground cumin, ground coriander, turmeric powder, and red chili powder. Cook for a minute to toast the spices, releasing their flavors.

4. Add Lentils and Tomatoes: Add the rinsed lentils and chopped tomatoes to the pot. Stir well to coat the lentils with the spices.

5. Add Water/Broth: Pour in the water or vegetable broth. You can adjust the amount of liquid based on how thick you want the curry to be.

6. Simmer: Bring the mixture to a boil, then reduce the heat to low. Cover the pot and let the lentils simmer for about 20-25 minutes, or until they are tender. Stir occasionally to prevent sticking.

7. Add Vegetables: Once the lentils are almost cooked, add the chopped mixed vegetables to the pot. Stir and let them cook for an additional 5-7 minutes, or until they are tender.

8. Season and Garnish: Add salt and garam masala to the curry. Taste and adjust the seasonings according to your preference. If you like it spicier, you can add more red chili powder.

9. Serve: Once the lentils and vegetables are cooked to your liking, remove the pot from heat. Garnish the curry with fresh cilantro leaves.

10. Enjoy: Serve the one-pot lentil curry hot with steamed rice, naan, or bread. The flavors will continue to develop as the curry sits, making it even more delicious the next day.

<u>One-pot lentil curry Prep Challenges and Solutions</u>

There are some potential problems you might encounter while preparing a one-pot lentil curry and their corresponding solutions:

<u>Problem 1: Lentils are too firm or undercooked</u>

Solution: If the lentils are not tender enough, continue simmering the curry for a few more minutes until they reach the desired consistency. You can also add a bit more water or broth if needed and continue cooking.

<u>Problem 2: Curry is too thin or watery</u>

Solution: If the curry turns out watery, remove the lid and let it simmer uncovered for a bit longer. This will allow excess moisture to evaporate and thicken the curry. You can also try mashing a small portion of the lentils with the back of a spoon to thicken the sauce.

<u>Problem 3: Curry is too thick</u>

Solution: If the curry becomes too thick, you can add a bit more water or broth to achieve the desired consistency. Remember to adjust the seasonings accordingly after adding more liquid.

Problem 4: Curry is too spicy

Solution: If the curry ends up spicier than you'd like, you can balance the heat by adding a squeeze of lemon or lime juice. You can also add a dollop of yogurt or a splash of coconut milk to mellow out the spiciness.

Problem 5: Vegetables are overcooked

Solution: If the vegetables become mushy, it's best to remove the curry from the heat immediately. While the curry may still be edible, the texture of the vegetables won't be ideal. To prevent this, add the vegetables later in the cooking process or choose vegetables that have a longer cooking time.

Problem 6: Lack of flavor

Solution: If the curry lacks flavor, consider adjusting the seasoning by adding more spices, salt, or even a dash of your favorite hot sauce. Taste and adjust until you achieve the desired flavor profile.

Problem 7: Burnt spices

Solution: Burnt spices can make the curry taste bitter. To prevent this, make sure to sauté the spices briefly and over low heat to avoid scorching. You can also add a bit of oil or liquid to the pot if you notice the spices sticking to the bottom.

Problem 8: Lentils are mushy

Solution: Overcooked lentils can become mushy and lose their texture. To avoid this, keep an eye on the lentils while they cook and test for doneness by tasting them periodically. Remove them from heat as soon as they are tender.

You can troubleshoot and adjust your cooking process to create a perfect one-pot lentil curry that's both delicious and satisfying by, being mindful of these potential issues and using the suggested solutions.

Rice and Vegetable Stir-Fry: A Delightful Fusion of Flavors

The sizzle of the wok, the aromatic medley of spices, and the colorful array of vegetables – these are the elements that come together in a rice and vegetable stir-fry, creating a dish that is not only visually appealing but also a delight for the taste buds. This culinary masterpiece has its roots in various Asian cuisines and has become a favorite across the globe due to its versatility and healthful qualities.

At the heart of a rice and vegetable stir-fry lies the harmony between rice and an assortment of fresh vegetables. The choice of vegetables is crucial, as it brings an array of textures, flavors, and nutrients to the dish. Bell peppers add a vibrant crunch, broccoli provides a subtle earthiness, carrots contribute sweetness, and snow peas lend a tender snap. This symphony of vegetables not only adds complexity to the dish but also ensures a well-rounded nutritional profile.

The process of creating a rice and vegetable stir-fry is an art in itself. It begins with preparing the vegetables – chopping, slicing, and dicing them into uniform sizes to ensure even cooking. The wok, a quintessential tool for this dish, is heated until it's almost smoking, and then a dash of oil is added, followed by aromatic ingredients like ginger and garlic. The kitchen is instantly filled with a delightful aroma that sets the stage for what's to come.

The vegetables are added next, each one introduced into the wok according to its cooking time, ensuring that none are overcooked or underdone. This precise choreography of ingredients highlights the chef's skill and attention to detail. Once the vegetables are slightly tender yet vibrant, cooked rice is added to the mix. The rice soaks up the flavors of the spices and vegetables, becoming a canvas upon which the symphony of tastes is painted.

The seasoning is where the magic truly happens. A delicate balance of soy sauce, oyster sauce, or other preferred sauces, combined with a sprinkle of spices and perhaps a hint of chili for those who prefer a touch of heat, brings the dish to life. The flavors meld together, creating a harmonious marriage of tastes that is at once savory, slightly salty, and subtly sweet.

The final result is a rice and vegetable stir-fry that is not only a treat for the senses but also a celebration of healthfulness. Packed with vitamins, minerals, and dietary fiber from the vegetables, and sustained energy from the rice, this dish satisfies both the palate and the body's nutritional needs.

Rice and vegetable stir-fry is a testament to the culinary prowess of blending flavors, textures, and colors. It transcends cultural boundaries, appealing to food enthusiasts worldwide. Whether enjoyed as a quick weeknight meal or presented with flair at a dinner party, this dish captures the essence of a wholesome and delectable fusion cuisine.

<u>Rice and Vegetable Stir-Fry Prep</u>

The itemized process for preparing Rice and Vegetable Stir-Fry are as follows:

<u>1. Gather Ingredients:</u>

- 2 cups of cooked rice (example quantity)
- Assorted vegetables (e.g., bell peppers, carrots, broccoli, snap peas)
- 1 tablespoon vegetable oil
- 2 cloves of garlic, minced
- 1 teaspoon ginger, minced
- Soy sauce (to taste)
- Salt and pepper (to taste)
- Optional: protein source (e.g., tofu, chicken, shrimp)

<u>2. Prep Vegetables:</u>

- Wash, peel (if needed), and chop the assorted vegetables into bite-sized pieces.

3. Cook Protein (if using):

- If using a protein source, cook it in a separate pan until fully cooked. Set aside.

4. Heat Oil:

- Heat the vegetable oil in a large pan or wok over medium-high heat.

5. Add Aromatics:

- Add minced garlic and ginger to the hot oil. Sauté for about 30 seconds until fragrant.

6. Stir-Fry Vegetables:

- Add the chopped vegetables to the pan. Stir-fry for 3-5 minutes until they start to become tender, but still have a slight crunch.

7. Seasoning:

- Season the vegetables with soy sauce, salt, and pepper. Adjust the quantities based on your taste preferences.

8. Add Cooked Rice:

- Add the cooked rice to the pan with the vegetables. Use a spatula to break up any clumps and mix everything.

9. Incorporate Protein (if using):

- If you prepared a protein source, add it to the pan and gently mix it with the rice and vegetables.

10. Stir-Fry:

- Continue stir-frying the mixture for another 2-3 minutes, allowing the flavors to meld and the rice to heat through.

11. Taste and Adjust:

- Taste the stir-fry and adjust the seasoning if needed. You can add more soy sauce or spices according to your preference.

12. Serve:

- Once everything is well combined and heated, remove the pan from the heat. Serve the Rice and Vegetable Stir-Fry in bowls or plates.

13. Garnish (Optional):

- Garnish with chopped green onions, sesame seeds, or a drizzle of sesame oil for extra flavor.

Rice and Vegetable Stir-Fry Prep Problems and Solutions

Some potential problems could arise during the preparation of Rice and Vegetable Stir-Fry, along with their corresponding solutions:

Problem 1: Overcooked Vegetables

- **Solution:** Be cautious not to overcook the vegetables. Keep an eye on them while stir-frying and remove from heat while they still have a slight crunch. This maintains their texture and flavor.

Problem 2: Underseasoned Dish

- **Solution:** Taste the stir-fry before serving and adjust the seasoning as needed. You can add more soy sauce, salt, or spices to enhance the flavors to your liking.

Problem 3: Sticky Rice

- **Solution:** If your rice becomes sticky while stir-frying, gently break up the clumps using a spatula. It's important to use pre-cooked and slightly cooled rice to prevent excessive stickiness.

Problem 4: Unbalanced Flavors

- **Solution:** To avoid unbalanced flavors, ensure that you use a suitable ratio of vegetables, rice, and protein. Additionally, consider the quantity of soy sauce and other seasonings to ensure a harmonious blend of flavors.

Problem 5: Burnt Aromatics

- **Solution:** Garlic and ginger can burn quickly. Keep the heat at a medium level and stir constantly while sautéing the aromatics. If they start to brown too quickly, lower the heat and add a splash of oil to prevent burning.

Problem 6: Overcrowded Pan

- **Solution:** If you overcrowd the pan with too many vegetables, they might not cook evenly. Consider stir-frying in batches or using a larger pan to ensure proper cooking.

Problem 7: Unevenly Cooked Protein

- **Solution:** If using a protein source like chicken or shrimp, make sure it's fully cooked before adding it to the stir-fry. Cook it separately if needed and add it to the dish towards the end, allowing it to warm through without overcooking.

Problem 8: Timing

- **Solution:** Timing is crucial in stir-frying. Prepare all ingredients ahead of time and have them ready to go. This helps ensure that you can quickly add ingredients to the pan without overcooking any element.

Pasta Primavera: A Symphony of Flavors and Colors

Pasta Primavera, a dish that encapsulates the essence of spring, is a delightful medley of fresh vegetables and pasta that dance harmoniously on the palate. This Italian-American creation has gained popularity for its vibrant colors, rich textures, and wholesome flavors.

As the winter frost melts away and nature awakens, Pasta Primavera makes its appearance, celebrating the abundance of seasonal vegetables. Bell peppers, carrots, zucchini, cherry tomatoes, and peas burst forth in a riot of hues, adding a visual feast to the plate. The vegetables are typically sautéed or lightly roasted, preserving their natural crispness and nutritional value.

Central to this dish is the pasta itself, often linguine or fettuccine, which provides a comforting canvas for the vegetable symphony. Cooked to al dente perfection, the pasta holds its own against the medley of vegetables, providing a satisfying texture that complements the crunch of the veggies.

The sauce that brings everything together is usually a simple amalgamation of olive oil, garlic, and sometimes a touch of cream or Parmesan cheese. This understated sauce allows the freshness of the vegetables to shine through, creating a balance between the richness of the pasta and the lightness of the produce.

Pasta Primavera is not just a culinary masterpiece; it's a representation of the changing seasons and a reminder of the beauty found in simplicity. It invites us to revel in the flavors nature offers, showcasing the bounties of the earth in a single, satisfying dish.

Pasta Primavera is more than just a meal; it's an ode to spring, a celebration of colors and flavors, and a testimony to the art of marrying simplicity with sophistication. As you savor each bite of this delightful dish, you're not just indulging your taste buds but also experiencing the rejuvenating spirit of the season on your plate.

<u>Pasta Primavera Prep</u>

An itemized process for preparing Pasta Primavera with random quantities for illustration is as follows:

<u>Ingredients:</u>

- 12 ounces of fettuccine pasta

- 1 red bell pepper

- 1 medium carrot

- 1 small zucchini

- 10 cherry tomatoes

- 1/2 cup of frozen peas

- 3 tablespoons of olive oil

- 3 cloves of garlic, minced

- Salt and pepper to taste

- 1/4 cup of heavy cream (optional)

- 1/4 cup of grated Parmesan cheese (optional)

- Fresh basil leaves for garnish

Instructions:

1. Boil the Pasta:

- Bring a pot of water (with a teaspoon of salt) to a boil.

- Add 12 ounces of fettuccine pasta and cook until al dente.

- Drain the pasta and set it aside.

2. Prepare the Vegetables:

- Wash and dice 1 red bell pepper, 1 medium carrot, and 1 small zucchini.

- Halve 10 cherry tomatoes.

- Measure 1/2 cup of frozen peas.

3. Sauté the Vegetables:

- In a large skillet, heat 3 tablespoons of olive oil over medium heat.

- Add 3 cloves of minced garlic and sauté for 1 minute until fragrant.

- Add the diced bell pepper, carrot, and zucchini. Sauté for 5-7 minutes until slightly tender.

4. Add Tomatoes and Peas:

- Add the halved cherry tomatoes and frozen peas to the skillet.

- Sauté for an additional 3-4 minutes until the tomatoes are slightly softened.

5. Prepare the Sauce:

- If using, pour 1/4 cup of heavy cream into the skillet.

- Optional: Add 1/4 cup of grated Parmesan cheese for extra flavor.

- Toss everything together to coat the vegetables with the cream and cheese. Let it simmer for 2 minutes.

6. Combine Pasta and Vegetables:

- Add the cooked fettuccine pasta to the skillet with the sautéed vegetables and sauce.

- Toss everything together to combine well.

7. Season and Garnish:

- Season the Pasta Primavera with salt and pepper to taste.

- Tear some fresh basil leaves and scatter them over the dish for a burst of freshness.

8. Serve:

- Divide the Pasta Primavera into serving plates.

- Enjoy the medley of flavors and colors in this delightful dish.

Pasta Primavera Prep Problems and Solutions

The potential problems that can arise during the preparation of Pasta Primavera and their corresponding solutions are as follows:

Problem 1: Overcooking Pasta

- If the pasta is cooked for too long, it can become mushy and lose its desired texture.

Solution: Properly Time Pasta Cooking

- Follow the package instructions for cooking time and test the pasta a couple of minutes before the suggested time to achieve the desired "al dente" texture.

- Have a timer set to avoid overcooking the pasta.

Problem 2: Unevenly Cooked Vegetables

- Vegetables may end up undercooked or overcooked if not prepared properly.

Solution: Uniform Chopping and Staggered Cooking

- Ensure vegetables are chopped into uniform sizes to promote even cooking.

- Add vegetables to the skillet in stages, starting with harder vegetables like carrots and gradually adding softer ones like tomatoes to prevent overcooking.

Problem 3: Insufficient Seasoning

- If the dish lacks proper seasoning, it can taste bland.

Solution: Season Gradually and Taste

- Season vegetables and pasta with salt and pepper in stages during the cooking process to layer flavors.

- Taste the dish as you go and adjust seasoning as needed.

Problem 4: Sauce Separation or Too Thick

- The sauce might separate or become too thick, affecting the overall consistency.

Solution: Use Emulsifiers and Adjust Thickness

- If using cream, slowly incorporate it while stirring to prevent separation.

- If the sauce becomes too thick, add a splash of pasta cooking water or extra olive oil to achieve the desired consistency.

Problem 5: Overwhelming the Dish with Ingredients

- Adding too many ingredients can lead to a crowded and chaotic dish.

Solution: Balance and Simplicity

- Limit the number of vegetables to maintain a balanced flavor and ensure each ingredient shines.

- Choose a few complementary vegetables and allow them to showcase their flavors.

Problem 6: Forgetting Freshness and Garnishes

- Neglecting to use of fresh herbs or garnishes can result in a less vibrant presentation.

Solution: Garnish and Elevate Presentation

- Sprinkle fresh herbs like basil or parsley over the finished dish for a burst of flavor and color.

- Consider adding a dash of lemon zest to brighten up the flavors.

<u>Exquisite Decadent Desserts</u>

Indulging in the world of desserts is a sensory delight that transcends culinary boundaries. From the first bite to the last, decadent desserts awaken our taste buds and offer a fleeting escape into a realm of pure pleasure. These luxurious treats, often rich in flavor and texture, hold the power to turn an ordinary moment into an extraordinary experience.

Imagine a velvety slice of chocolate truffle cake, its deep cocoa aroma enveloping you as you delve into its luscious layers. Each bite is a symphony of smoothness and intensity, leaving behind a hint of bittersweet ecstasy that lingers on the palate. Such desserts are not merely confections; they are works of art, carefully crafted to evoke emotions and trigger memories.

Decadent desserts go beyond their taste; they are an embodiment of creativity and craftsmanship. Take, for instance, the delicate artistry of a fruit-topped cheesecake. The creaminess of the cheese filling juxtaposed with the tartness of berries creates a harmonious dance of flavors that delights both the senses and the soul. The presentation, too, is a feast for the eyes, with vibrant colors and intricate designs that mirror the chef's dedication.

These indulgent creations often transcend cultural boundaries, finding their way onto menus around the world. Tiramisu, a classic Italian delight, layers coffee-soaked ladyfingers with mascarpone cheese, resulting in a dessert that is simultaneously bold and comforting. On the other side of the globe, the French macaron captivates with its delicate meringue shells and exquisite fillings, showcasing the finesse of French patisserie.

However, the allure of decadent desserts is not solely reserved for those with a sweet tooth. They provide an avenue for innovation, allowing chefs to experiment with unexpected combinations of flavors and textures. Salted caramel brownies, for instance, balance the sugary sweetness of caramel with a touch of saltiness, creating a mesmerizing contrast that keeps the taste buds intrigued.

In a world where culinary experiences are cherished, decadent desserts hold a special place. They mark celebrations, symbolize love, and offer comfort in times of need. Whether it's a towering slice of layered cake, a delicate pastry, or a scoop of artisanal ice cream, these desserts invite us to savor the moment, appreciating the skill and passion that go into their creation. So, the next time you find yourself in the presence of a decadent dessert, take a moment to relish not just its taste, but the stories and emotions it carries, making life a little sweeter with each delectable bite.

<u>Exquisite Decadent Desserts Problems and Solutions</u>

There are common problems that might arise during the preparation of decadent desserts, along with their solutions:

<u>Problem 1: Cake is Dry</u>

- **Cause:** Overbaking the cake can lead to dryness.

- **Solution:** To prevent this, monitor the baking time closely and perform a toothpick test. Insert a toothpick into the center of the cake; if it comes out clean or with a few moist crumbs, the cake is done.

<u>Problem 2: Mousse Doesn't Set Properly</u>

- **Cause:** If the mousse doesn't set, it might be due to incorrect proportions of ingredients or not allowing enough chilling time.

- **Solution:** Ensure you're using the correct ingredient ratios and follow the recipe closely. Refrigerate the dessert for the recommended time, often several hours or overnight, to allow the mousse to be properly set.

Problem 3: Chocolate Seizes

- **Cause:** Chocolate can seize when it comes into contact with water or if it's overheated.

- **Solution:** Melt the chocolate slowly using a double boiler or microwave in short bursts, stirring between each burst. Avoid adding water to melted chocolate. If chocolate seizes, you can try adding a small amount of warm milk or cream and gently stirring until smooth.

Problem 4: Cake Doesn't Release from Pan

- **Cause:** If the cake sticks to the pan, it can break apart when trying to remove it.

- **Solution:** Make sure to properly grease and line the cake pan before pouring in the batter. Allow the cake to cool slightly before attempting to remove it from the pan.

Problem 5: Whipped Cream Won't Whip

- **Cause:** Factors like low-fat content or over-whipping can prevent the cream from whipping properly.

- **Solution:** Use heavy cream with a high fat content (around 36%). Chill the cream, bowl, and beaters before whipping. Whip until soft peaks form; over-whipped cream can turn into butter.

Problem 6: Mousse Layers Mix

- **Cause:** If the mousse layers blend, it might be due to improper chilling or pouring.

- **Solution:** Allow each mousse layer to set properly before adding the next layer. Pour the mousse gently over the cake layer using a spatula to create a barrier between the layers.

Problem 7: Overwhelming Flavors

- **Cause:** Overusing strong flavors or not balancing flavors can result in an overwhelming taste.

- **Solution:** Use flavors sparingly and consider the balance between sweet, bitter, and tart elements. Taste as you go and adjust ingredients accordingly.

Problem 8: Decorations Don't Stay in Place

- **Cause:** Decorations like berries or grated chocolate can slide off the dessert.

- **Solution:** After placing decorations on the dessert, gently press them in place. You can also use a small amount of softened chocolate as "glue" to hold decorations.

Chocolate Raspberry Mousse Cake Prep

This is a breakdown of the process of preparing a decadent dessert, a "Chocolate Raspberry Mousse Cake".

Ingredients:

- 200g dark chocolate

- 150g fresh raspberries

- 250g heavy cream

- 100g granulated sugar

- 3 large eggs

- 1 teaspoon vanilla extract

- 150g all-purpose flour

- 1 teaspoon baking powder

- Pinch of salt

Process:

1. Preheat the Oven:

Preheat your oven to 350°F (175°C).

2. Prepare the Cake:

- In a mixing bowl, whisk 2 eggs and 50g of sugar until light and fluffy.

- Melt 100g of dark chocolate and fold it into the egg mixture.

- Sift in 150g of flour, baking powder, and a pinch of salt. Gently fold until just combined.

- Pour the batter into a greased and lined cake pan.

- Bake for 20-25 minutes or until a toothpick comes out clean. Let it cool.

3. Prepare the Raspberry Mousse:

- Puree 100g of raspberries in a blender and strain to remove seeds.

- Whip 150g of heavy cream until soft peaks form.

- Gently fold the raspberry puree into the whipped cream.

4. Prepare the Chocolate Mousse:

- Melt 100g of dark chocolate and let it cool slightly.

- Separate the remaining egg yolk and egg white.

- In a heatproof bowl, whisk together the egg yolk and 50g of sugar. Place it over a pot of simmering water and whisk until it thickens.

- Remove from heat, add melted chocolate and vanilla extract. Mix well.

- Whip the remaining 100g of heavy cream until soft peaks form. Fold it into the chocolate mixture.

5. Assemble the Cake:

- Cut the cooled cake into two layers.

- Place one layer of cake at the bottom of a cake ring or springform pan.

- Spread a layer of raspberry mousse over the cake layer.

- Add a second layer of cake on top and gently press down.

- Pour the chocolate mousse over the cake layer.

- Refrigerate for at least 4 hours, preferably overnight, to allow the mousse to set.

6. Decorate and Serve:

- Carefully remove the cake ring or springform pan.

- Decorate the top with fresh raspberries and some grated chocolate.

- Slice and serve this delightful chocolate raspberry mousse cake, savoring each decadent bite.

<u>Chocolate Raspberry Mousse Cake Prep</u>
<u>Problems and Solutions</u>

Problems:

1. Curled Chocolate Decorations: Chocolate decorations can curl or break during the process.

Solution: Handle the chocolate decorations gently and work in a cool room to avoid melting. Properly temper the chocolate to improve its stability.

2. Soggy Cake Layers: Moisture from the mousse can make the cake layers soggy.

Solution: Brush the cake layers with a thin layer of melted chocolate or simple syrup to create a barrier that prevents moisture from seeping in.

3. Mousse Doesn't Set: The mousse may not set properly, leading to a runny texture.

Solution: Make sure to properly whip the heavy cream and fold it into the chocolate mixture gently. Additionally, ensure you're using the right proportion of gelatin to help the mousse set.

4. Air Bubbles in Mousse: Air bubbles can create an uneven texture in the mousse.

Solution: Gently fold the whipped cream into the chocolate mixture in a slow, deliberate motion. Avoid overmixing to prevent excessive incorporation of air.

5. Uneven Layers: Assembling the cake with uneven layers can affect its appearance and stability.

Solution: Use a cake leveler to ensure each layer is even in thickness. Take your time when stacking the layers and apply the mousse evenly between them.

6. Raspberries Release Moisture: Raspberries can release moisture and cause the cake to become soggy.

Solution: Place a thin layer of mousse between the raspberries and the cake layers to create a moisture barrier. You can also use freeze-dried raspberries to add flavor without excess moisture.

7. Difficulty in Unmolding: The cake might stick to the sides of the mold, making it difficult to unmold.

Solution: Line the mold with acetate strips or parchment paper to create an easy-release surface. Chilling the cake for a longer period before attempting to unmold can also help.

8. Ganache Issues: The ganache for the glaze might be too thick or too thin.

Solution: Adjust the ganache consistency by either adding more cream to thin it out or adding more chocolate to thicken it. Test the ganache on a small area of the cake to ensure the desired consistency is achieved

Chocolate Avocado Mousse Prep

Itemized processes for preparing Chocolate Avocado Mousse are as follows:

1. Ingredients:

- Avocado (1 large or 2 small)

- Dark chocolate (about 100g)

- Sweetener (such as honey, maple syrup, or agave), to taste

- Cocoa powder (2-3 tablespoons)

- Vanilla extract (1 teaspoon)

- Pinch of salt

- Optional toppings: whipped cream, berries, nuts

2. Preparation:

a. Melt Chocolate:

- Break the dark chocolate into small pieces and melt it using a microwave or double boiler method. Let it cool slightly.

b. Prepare Avocado:

- Cut the avocado(s) in half, remove the pit, and scoop out the flesh.

c. Blend Ingredients:

- In a food processor or blender, combine the avocado, melted chocolate, sweetener, cocoa powder, vanilla extract, and a pinch of salt.

- Blend until smooth and creamy. Taste and adjust sweetness if needed.

d. Adjust Consistency:

- If the mixture is too thick, you can add a splash of milk (dairy or non-dairy) to achieve the desired consistency.

e. Chill:

- Transfer the mixture to serving dishes or glasses.

f. Refrigerate:

- Cover the dishes with plastic wrap or lids and refrigerate the mousse for at least 1-2 hours to allow it to set and the flavors to meld.

g. Serve:

- Once chilled, remove the mousse from the refrigerator.

- Optionally, top with whipped cream, berries, nuts, or any other desired toppings before serving.

Know that ingredients can vary based on your preferences, so feel free to adjust them according to taste.

<u>Chocolate Avocado Mousse Prep Problems and Solutions</u>

Potential problems you might encounter while preparing Chocolate Avocado Mousse and their corresponding solutions:

Problem: Mousse is too bitter

- **Solution:** Add more sweetener (honey, maple syrup, or agave) to balance the bitterness of the cocoa and avocado. Blend and taste until the desired level of sweetness is achieved.

<u>Problem: Mousse is too thick</u>

- **Solution:** Gradually add a small amount of milk (dairy or non-dairy) to the mixture while blending until you reach the desired consistency. Be cautious not to make it too runny.

Problem: The avocado flavor is too strong

- **Solution:** Increase the amount of cocoa powder and/or sweetener to mask the avocado taste. You can also try adding a bit more vanilla extract for a stronger flavor profile.

Problem: Mousse is not creamy enough

- **Solution:** Ensure that the avocado is fully ripe and soft before using. Blend the mixture thoroughly until it's completely smooth and creamy. You can also adjust the sweetener and chocolate to improve the texture.

Problem: Mousse doesn't set properly

- **Solution:** Make sure to refrigerate the mousse for the recommended time (at least 1-2 hours) to allow it to set. If the mousse is still too soft, you can blend in a small amount of melted and cooled dark chocolate to help it firm up.

Problem: Mousse has an unpleasant aftertaste

- **Solution:** Ensure that all the ingredients are of good quality and fresh. If the mousse has an aftertaste, it could be due to the quality of the chocolate, avocado, or sweetener used.

Problem: Texture is lumpy or grainy

- **Solution:** To achieve a smooth texture, blend the mixture thoroughly in a food processor or blender. If you're using a blender, you might need to stop and scrape down the sides to ensure everything is well combined.

Cooking and baking often involve some trial and error, don't be discouraged by minor setbacks. Adjusting ingredients and techniques can help you achieve the perfect Chocolate Avocado Mousse you're aiming for.

<u>Berry Parfait with Almond Crumble</u>

Berry Parfait with Almond Crumble is a delightful and versatile dessert that brings together a medley of flavors and textures to create a truly enjoyable culinary experience. This exquisite dessert combines the natural sweetness of fresh berries with the nutty crunch of almond crumble, resulting in a harmonious blend of taste and texture that is sure to delight the palate.

One of the key attributes of this dessert is its visual appeal. The vibrant colors of the assorted berries create an enticing presentation that is not only visually pleasing but also indicative of the dish's nutritional value. Berries are renowned for their high antioxidant content, which can contribute to overall well-being and support a healthy immune system.

The contrast between the creamy layers of parfait and the crisp almond crumble adds a delightful complexity to each bite. The smoothness of the parfait provides a soothing backdrop for the burst of flavors from the berries, while the almond crumble introduces a satisfying element of crunchiness. This combination of textures elevates the dessert beyond a simple sweet treat, making it an experience that engages both the senses and the taste buds.

Moreover, the "Berry Parfait with Almond Crumble" offers a balanced combination of indulgence and nutritional value. While the parfait offers a creamy and indulgent base, the inclusion of fresh berries ensures a dose of vitamins, minerals, and dietary fiber. The almond crumble not only adds a delectable nutty flavor but also contributes healthy fats and additional crunch, making this dessert a more wholesome option compared to many other sugary treats.

Whether enjoyed as a light post-meal dessert or as a standalone snack, the "Berry Parfait with Almond

Crumble" serves as a versatile choice suitable for various occasions. Its elegant presentation makes it fitting for formal gatherings, while its wholesome ingredients make it an option that can align with health-conscious preferences.

In conclusion, the "Berry Parfait with Almond Crumble" stands out as a culinary masterpiece that marries taste, texture, and nutritional value in a single dish. Its versatility, visual appeal, and harmonious blend of flavors and textures make it a delightful addition to any menu. Whether you're looking for a treat that indulges your senses or a dessert that nourishes your body, this parfait is a perfect choice that showcases the artistry and creativity of modern gastronomy.

<u>Berry Parfait with Almond Crumble Prep</u>

This is an itemized process for preparing Berry Parfait with Almond Crumble with random quantity of ingredients:

<u>Ingredients:</u>

- 1 cup mixed fresh berries (strawberries, blueberries, raspberries)
- 1 cup Greek yogurt
- 1/4 cup granola
- 1/4 cup sliced almonds
- 2 tablespoons honey
- 1 teaspoon vanilla extract

<u>Almond Crumble:</u>

1. Preheat the oven to 350°F (175°C).
2. In a mixing bowl, combine 1/4 cup of sliced almonds with 1 tablespoon of honey and a pinch of salt.

3. Spread the almond mixture evenly on a baking sheet and bake for about 8-10 minutes, or until the almonds are golden and toasted. Allow to cool.

Berry Compote:

1. In a saucepan, add 1/2 cup of mixed berries, 1 tablespoon of honey, and 1 teaspoon of vanilla extract.
2. Cook the mixture over medium heat, stirring occasionally, until the berries break down and the mixture thickens slightly. Remove from heat and let it cool.

Assembling the Parfait:

1. In serving glasses or bowls, start by layering 2 tablespoons of Greek yogurt at the bottom.

2. Add a spoonful of the berry compote on top of the yogurt layer.

3. Sprinkle a teaspoon of granola over the compote.

4. Drizzle a bit of honey over the granola layer.

5. Repeat the layers with yogurt, compote, granola, and honey until the glass is filled, finishing with a layer of berries on top.

Final Assembly:

1. Just before serving, sprinkle the cooled almond crumble over the top layer of berries.

2. Optionally, garnish with a few fresh mint leaves for added freshness.

Serve the "Berry Parfait with Almond Crumble" immediately to enjoy the contrast of textures and flavors.

<u>Berry Parfait with Almond Crumble Problems and Solutions</u>

These are itemized lists of potential problems that might arise during the preparation of Berry Parfait with Almond Crumble, along with their corresponding solutions, by being aware of these potential issues and having the corresponding solutions in mind, you can confidently prepare a delicious and visually appealing "Berry Parfait with Almond Crumble" while minimizing any hiccups along the way.

<u>Problem: Berries are not fresh or are overripe.</u>

Solution: Choose fresh and ripe berries. Wash and dry them properly before use. If berries are overripe, consider using them for the berry compote to salvage their flavor.

<u>Problem: Almond crumble burns in the oven.</u>

Solution: Keep a close eye on the almonds while toasting and set a timer to prevent over-baking. Stir the almonds halfway through baking to ensure even toasting.

Problem: Greek yogurt is too thick to layer easily.

Solution: You can loosen the Greek yogurt by stirring in a small amount of milk or cream to achieve a smoother consistency for layering.

Problem: Berry's compote turns out too runny.

Solution: If the compote is too runny, return it to the heat and simmer for a few more minutes until it thickens. You can also add a bit of cornstarch mixed with water as a thickening agent.

Problem: Parfait layers are not visually distinct.

Solution: To achieve clear and visually appealing layers, use a piping bag or a zip-top bag with a corner snipped off to add the yogurt, compote, and granola layers neatly.

Problem: Granola becomes soggy from contact with yogurt.

Solution: To prevent granola from becoming soggy, consider adding it just before serving. Alternatively, you can layer the granola on top of the yogurt layers to maintain its crunchiness.

Problem: Parfait tastes too sweet.

Solution: Adjust the amount of honey used in each layer to suit your taste. You can also choose to use unsweetened Greek yogurt and reduce the amount of honey in the berry compote.

Problem: Not enough almond crumble for the desired number of servings.

Solution: Ensure you prepare enough almond crumble to accommodate the number of servings you plan to make. If you run short, you can quickly prepare more almond crumble using the same method.

<u>Energy-Packed Date-Nut Balls</u>

In today's fast-paced world, finding healthy and convenient snacks is essential. One such delightful option that has gained popularity is the "Date and Nut Energy Balls." These small, power-packed treats are not only delicious but also offer a plethora of nutritional benefits.

Comprising mainly dates and various nuts, these energy balls are a rich source of natural energy. Dates, with their natural sugars, provide an instant energy boost, while nuts like almonds, walnuts, and cashews offer healthy fats, protein, and essential minerals. This combination makes these energy balls an ideal choice for a quick pre-or post-workout snack or a mid-afternoon pick-me-up.

The preparation of date and nut energy balls is simple and customizable. Typically, the ingredients are blended into a sticky mixture, which is then rolled into bite-sized balls. Creative variations abound, as one can add ingredients like chia seeds, coconut flakes, cocoa powder, or even a hint of natural sweeteners like honey or maple syrup. This adaptability ensures that there's a flavor combination to suit every palate.

What sets these energy balls apart is not just their taste, but their nutritional value. They are an excellent source of dietary fiber, aiding digestion and promoting a feeling of fullness. The nuts in these balls provide heart-healthy fats and essential nutrients like vitamin E and magnesium. Moreover, they are a great alternative to sugary snacks, contributing to better weight management and blood sugar control.

For those with dietary restrictions, date, and nut energy balls are a blessing. They are naturally gluten-free and can be easily adapted to suit vegan diets. These qualities make them a go-to option for individuals looking for allergy-friendly, nutrient-dense snacks.

In conclusion, date and nut energy balls are a delicious and nutritious snack option that aligns perfectly with today's health-conscious lifestyle. Whether you need a quick energy boost, a satisfying post-workout bite, or simply a tasty treat that won't compromise your health goals, these energy balls have got you covered. With their simplicity of preparation and versatility in flavors, they are a wonderful addition to anyone's culinary repertoire.

<u>Energy-Packed Date-Nut Balls Prep</u>

Here's an itemized process for preparing Energy-Packed Date-Nut Balls, with a random quantity example:

<u>Ingredients:</u>

- 1 cup pitted dates

- 1/2 cup mixed nuts (almonds and walnuts)

- 1/2 cup rolled oats

- 1/4 cup almond butter

- 2 tablespoons honey

- 2 tablespoons cocoa powder

- 1 teaspoon vanilla extract

- Coconut flakes (for rolling)

<u>Instructions:</u>

<u>1. Blend Nuts and Oats:</u>

- In a food processor, blend 1/2 cup mixed nuts and 1/2 cup rolled oats until coarse.

2. Add Dates:

- Add 1 cup pitted dates to the nut and oat mixture. Blend until well combined.

3. Add Almond Butter and Honey:

- Add 1/4 cup almond butter and 2 tablespoons honey to the mixture. Blend until it forms a sticky dough.

4. Incorporate Cocoa and Vanilla:

- Add 2 tablespoons cocoa powder and 1 teaspoon vanilla extract. Blend until the mixture is evenly chocolaty.

5. Check Consistency:

- Test the mixture by rolling a small amount into a ball. If it holds shape, it's ready. Otherwise, add a bit more almond butter.

6. Form Balls:

- Take spoonfuls of the mixture and roll into bite-sized balls. This should yield around 12 balls.

7. Roll in Coconut Flakes:

- Roll each ball in coconut flakes, pressing gently to adhere.

8. Chill and Set:

- Place the balls on a parchment-lined tray and refrigerate for at least 30 minutes to firm up.

9. Store:

- Once set, transfer the balls to an airtight container and store in the refrigerator.

10. Enjoy:

- Your Energy-Packed Date-Nut Balls are ready to enjoy! Grab them as a nutritious snack anytime.

Quantities and ingredients are adjustable according to your taste and preferences.

Energy-Packed Date-Nut Balls Prep Problems and Solutions

The potential problems you might encounter while preparing Energy-Packed Date-Nut Balls, along with their solutions:

Problem 1: Mixture is Too Dry

- If the mixture doesn't stick together well and feels too dry, the balls won't hold their shape.

Solution:

- Add a bit more nut butter (e.g., almond butter) or a touch of honey to the mixture. Blend again until the mixture becomes stickier and holds together when pressed.

Problem 2: Mixture is Too Sticky

- On the other hand, if the mixture is overly sticky, it might be difficult to form neat balls.

Solution:

- Incorporate more rolled oats or ground nuts to balance out the stickiness. This will help you achieve the desired consistency for rolling.

Problem 3: Balls Won't Hold Shape

- If the formed balls aren't holding their shape and are falling apart, it could be due to the mixture being too loose.

Solution:

- Add more nut butter, honey, or dates to bind the mixture better. Alternatively, consider adding ground nuts or oats to give the mixture more structure.

Problem 4: Flavor Isn't Balanced

- The flavor might be too sweet, not sweet enough, or lacking in other desired flavors.

Solution:

- Taste the mixture before forming balls. If it's too sweet, consider reducing the amount of sweetener or adding more nuts and oats. For more flavor, adjust the cocoa powder, vanilla extract, or other flavorings to your preference.

Problem 5: Balls are Falling Apart While Rolling

- If the balls are breaking apart while you're trying to roll them, it might be due to the mixture not being well-combined.

Solution:

- Ensure that the ingredients are blended thoroughly in the food processor. Also, press the mixture firmly while rolling to help it hold its shape.

Problem 6: Balls are Too Large or Too Small

- If the size of the balls isn't consistent, it can affect the overall presentation and texture.

<u>Solution:</u>

- Use a measuring spoon or scoop to portion out the mixture, ensuring that each portion is of similar size. This will help you achieve consistent balls.

Don't be afraid to experiment and adapt the recipe to suit your preferences and avoid common pitfalls. Understand that making adjustments while preparing the mixture is key to achieving the right consistency and flavor.

Kitchen Staples

In every culinary endeavor, from a simple weeknight dinner to an elaborate feast, the role of kitchen staples cannot be overstated. These essential ingredients form the foundation upon which culinary creations are built, offering both convenience and versatility to home cooks and professional chefs alike.

At the heart of any kitchen lies a well-stocked pantry, brimming with staples that transform the ordinary into the extraordinary. Flour, sugar, and baking powder come together to craft the perfect cake; rice, pasta, and beans offer sustenance in various forms; and a spectrum of oils and vinegars add depth and complexity to dishes. These ingredients transcend cultural boundaries and enable cooks to explore a plethora of cuisines from around the world.

Herbs and spices, another category of kitchen staples, possess the power to elevate dishes to new heights. A pinch of aromatic basil, a dash of pungent cumin, or a sprinkle of fiery red pepper flakes can awaken the senses and turn a simple dish into a culinary masterpiece. These flavor enhancers not only add taste but also contribute to the visual appeal of the final presentation.

Canned goods, such as tomatoes, broth, and coconut milk, offer convenience without compromising taste. They provide a backup plan when fresh ingredients are scarce or out of season, ensuring that home-cooked meals are never far from reach. And while fresh produce is revered for its nutritional value, frozen fruits and vegetables are invaluable staples that retain their nutrients while being available year-round.

Dairy products like milk, eggs, and butter are the unsung heroes of countless recipes, from scrambled eggs to creamy sauces. Their ability to bind, emulsify, and add richness to dishes makes them indispensable in the kitchen. Similarly, condiments like mustard, ketchup, and mayonnaise inject a burst of flavor and can be used to create a myriad of sauces and dressings.

In recent times, as culinary preferences evolve, dietary restrictions are considered, and global ingredients become more accessible, the definition of kitchen staples has expanded. Non-dairy milk alternatives, gluten-free flours, and plant-based proteins now take their place alongside traditional staples, catering to a diverse range of tastes and needs.

In conclusion, kitchen staples are the cornerstone of culinary creativity and convenience. They empower cooks to experiment, innovate, and create memorable dishes, all while providing a safety net of ingredients to fall back on. A well-curated collection of pantry essentials not only saves time and effort but also ensures that the joy of cooking is always within reach, transforming the everyday act of preparing meals into an art form.

The list of common kitchen staples are as follows:

1. Salt

2. Pepper

3. Olive oil

4. Vinegar (such as balsamic or white vinegar)

5. All-purpose flour

6. Sugar (granulated and brown)

7. Rice

8. Pasta

9. Canned tomatoes

10. Onions

11. Garlic

12. Butter

13. Eggs

14. Milk

15. Bread

16. Spices (such as oregano, thyme, cumin, and paprika)

17. Stock or broth (chicken, vegetable, or beef)

18. Soy sauce

19. Honey

20. Mustard

This list can vary depending on your cooking preferences, but these are some common items found in many kitchens.

Homemade Nut Butter Prep

Let's go through the process of preparing homemade nut butter with a random quantity of 2 cups of almonds:

1. Ingredients:

- 2 cups of almonds

- Pinch of salt (optional)

- 1 tablespoon of honey (optional)

- 1 teaspoon of vanilla extract (optional)

- 2 tablespoons of neutral oil (if needed)

2. Roasting (Optional):

- Preheat the oven to 350°F (175°C).

- Spread 2 cups of almonds on a baking sheet and roast for about 12 minutes until they're slightly golden and fragrant.

- Allow the roasted almonds to cool for a few minutes.

3. Blending:

- Transfer the roasted almonds to a high-powered food processor.

- Add a pinch of salt, 1 tablespoon of honey, and 1 teaspoon of vanilla extract if desired.

4. Start Blending:

- Begin blending the almonds on low speed. The nuts will break down into a coarse powder.

5. Scraping:

- Pause the blending and scrape down the sides of the container to ensure even blending.

6. Blending Continues:

- Continue blending on low to medium speed. The mixture will start to clump together and become sticky.

7. Achieving Creaminess:

- Keep blending until the almonds release their natural oils and the mixture turns creamy. This might take several minutes.

8. Adjust Consistency:

- If the nut butter seems too thick, add 2 tablespoons of neutral oil to achieve the desired consistency. Blend again to combine.

9. Taste and Adjust:

- Taste the nut butter and adjust the flavor by adding more salt, honey, or vanilla extract if needed.

10. Storage:

- Transfer the homemade almond butter to a clean, airtight jar.

- Store it in the refrigerator and give it a good stir before each use.

You can adjust these quantities and ingredients based on your preferences and the available ingredients.

Homemade Nut Butter Prep Problems and Solutions

Problem 1: Nut Butter Too Thick

- **Solution:** Add a small amount of neutral oil, such as peanut or coconut oil, to the mixture while blending. This will help achieve a smoother and more spreadable consistency.

Problem 2: Nut Butter Too Thin or Runny

- **Solution:** If you've added too much oil or the nut butter is too thin, you can thicken it by incorporating additional nuts. Blend in small amounts of nuts at a time until the desired consistency is reached.

Problem 3: Nut Butter Not Creamy

- **Solution:** Achieving a creamy texture can take time. Continue blending the nuts until they release their natural oils and the mixture becomes smooth. Be patient and give the food processor breaks if needed.

Problem 4: Overheating the Blender/Food Processor

- **Solution:** If your blender or food processor starts to get too hot during blending, pause and allow it to cool down before continuing. Overheating can affect the texture and quality of the nut butter.

Problem 5: Nut Butter Separation

- **Solution:** It's normal for nut butter to separate a bit over time, with oil rising to the top. Before using, simply give the nut butter a good stir to recombine the oils and solids.

Problem 6: Over-Processing

- **Solution:** Avoid over-processing the nut butter, as this can cause the oils to separate and make the texture grainy. Stop blending once you've achieved the desired creamy consistency.

Problem 7: Allergies

- **Solution:** Be cautious of any allergies you or others might have to nuts or other ingredients used in the nut butter. Always label your homemade nut butter with its ingredients in case others will be consuming it.

This process might require some experimentation to get the nut butter exactly how you like it. Don't be afraid to adjust ingredients and quantities as needed to achieve your desired flavor and texture.

<u>Crafting Flavorful Delights with DIY No-Salt Seasoning Blends</u>

In a world where health-conscious choices are becoming increasingly vital, the quest to create delectable dishes while maintaining a balanced diet has led to the rise of the DIY no-salt seasoning blend. This innovative culinary approach not only tantalizes taste buds but also champions wellness by reducing sodium intake without compromising on flavor.

Salt has long been a staple in kitchens, enhancing flavors and preserving foods. However, as health concerns mount, the spotlight has shifted towards finding healthier alternatives. The DIY no-salt seasoning blend emerges as a creative solution, transforming the art of seasoning into a harmonious symphony of herbs, spices, and aromatic ingredients.

Crafting your personalized no-salt blend is an adventure in itself. Begin by selecting a medley of dried herbs – basil, thyme, oregano, or rosemary – each bringing its unique essence to the mix. These botanical wonders infuse dishes with depth and character. Complementing the herbs are a selection of spices like robust paprika, zesty black pepper, and the warmth of cumin. Together, they dance on the palate, creating a sensation that salt alone could never replicate.

The canvas of flavor isn't complete without the addition of piquant garlic and onion powders. These allies add a savory touch, establishing a savory foundation that elevates the dish. For those seeking a touch of vibrancy, a sprinkle of citrus zest – lemon, lime, or orange – introduces a burst of freshness, offering a symphony of taste that awakens the senses.

The beauty of the DIY no-salt seasoning blend lies in its versatility. From grilled vegetables to roasted meats, soups, and even salads, this blend seamlessly integrates into various culinary creations. A mere pinch can transform mundane ingredients into a culinary masterpiece that delights both the palate and the body.

Beyond its culinary prowess, the DIY no-salt seasoning blend paves the way for healthier living. By curbing excessive sodium consumption, it supports cardiovascular health and aids in managing blood pressure. Moreover, it encourages culinary experimentation, inspiring individuals to explore new avenues of flavor, discover hidden tastes, and embrace the art of mindful cooking.

The DIY no-salt seasoning blend is more than a mere kitchen experiment; it is a flavorful revolution that empowers individuals to make conscious choices without sacrificing taste. As we embrace this gastronomic journey, we redefine the way we season our lives – with vibrancy, creativity, and a dash of wellness. So, let the concoction of herbs and spices be the palette with which you paint your culinary masterpiece, crafting a healthier and more flavorful world, one dish at a time.

DIY No-Salt Seasoning Blends Prep

1. Gather Ingredients:

Collect various dried herbs and spices such as garlic powder, onion powder, black pepper, paprika, thyme, oregano, rosemary, and any other seasonings you prefer.

2. Choose a Recipe:

Look up a DIY no-salt seasoning blend recipe online or create your own based on your taste preferences. Make sure to include a variety of herbs and spices.

3. Select a Quantity:

Choose a random quantity for your seasoning blend. Let's say you decide on making a batch that fills a small spice jar (approximately 1/4 cup).

4. Calculate Measurements:

Adjust the quantities of each ingredient in the recipe to match the chosen quantity. If the recipe serves 1 cup and you're making 1/4 cup, divide all ingredient measurements by 4.

5. Prepare Ingredients:

Measure out the herbs and spices according to your adjusted recipe. Use measuring spoons for accurate amounts.

6. Mix Thoroughly:

In a small bowl, combine all the measured ingredients. Stir or whisk well to ensure an even distribution of flavors.

7. Taste and Adjust:

Take a small sample of the seasoning blend and taste it. Adjust the quantities of specific ingredients if necessary to achieve the desired flavor balance.

8. Store in a Container:

Transfer the seasoning blend to an airtight container, such as a spice jar or a small glass container. Make sure the container is clean and dry.

9. Label the Container:

Create a label for the container indicating the name of the seasoning blend, the date it was made, and any additional information you'd like to include.

10. Store in a Cool Place:

Keep the container in a cool, dry, and dark place to preserve the flavors of the seasoning blend. Avoid exposing it to direct sunlight or heat.

11. Use in Cooking:

Incorporate your DIY no-salt seasoning blend into various dishes as a flavorful substitute for salt.

Experiment with different recipes to enjoy its taste-enhancing qualities.

Oil-free Salad Dressing Prep

The process for preparing an oil-free salad dressing with a random ingredients quantity are as follows:

1. Gather Ingredients: Collect your chosen ingredients. For example, let's consider a sample quantity for a single serving:

- 2 tablespoons of balsamic vinegar

- 1 tablespoon of Dijon mustard

- 1 clove of garlic (minced)

- 1 teaspoon of maple syrup

- Salt and pepper to taste

- Chopped fresh herbs (optional)

2. Mix Vinegar and Mustard: In a mixing bowl, combine 2 tablespoons of balsamic vinegar and 1 tablespoon of Dijon mustard.

3. Add Garlic and Maple Syrup: Add the minced clove of garlic and 1 teaspoon of maple syrup to the bowl. Mix well to combine the flavors.

4. Season: Sprinkle in a pinch of salt and pepper to taste. You can adjust the amount according to your preference.

5. Incorporate Herbs: If desired, add a tablespoon of chopped fresh herbs like basil, thyme, or parsley. This can enhance the aroma and taste of the dressing.

6. Whisk or Shake: Whisk the mixture vigorously or place all the ingredients in a sealed container and shake it until everything is well combined.

7. Taste and Adjust: Taste a small amount of the dressing and adjust the flavors as needed. You can add more vinegar, mustard, sweetener, or seasoning to balance the taste to your liking.

8. Serve: Your oil-free salad dressing is ready to use. Drizzle it over your favorite salad ingredients and toss to coat.

You can experiment with different vinegars, herbs, and seasonings to create variations that suit your taste preferences.

Oil-free Salad Dressing Prep Problems And Solutions

Problem 1: Too Tangy or Acidic Flavor

- **Issue:** The dressing might turn out too tangy or acidic due to the vinegar.

- **Solution:** To balance the flavors, you can add a bit more maple syrup to add sweetness. Alternatively, you can dilute the dressing with a small amount of water or a non-dairy milk like almond milk to mellow out the acidity.

Problem 2: Bland or Lacking Depth of Flavor

- **Issue:** The dressing might lack complexity and depth of flavor.

- **Solution:** Consider adding more minced garlic for a stronger savory taste. You can also experiment with additional herbs and spices, such as dried oregano, basil, or a pinch of red pepper flakes, to enhance the overall flavor profile.

Problem 3: Separation of Ingredients

- **Issue:** The ingredients might not emulsify properly, causing separation.

- **Solution:** Emulsify the dressing more effectively by using a blender or a handheld immersion blender. This will create a smoother and more cohesive texture. Additionally, shaking the dressing vigorously in a sealed container before each use can help prevent separation.

Problem 4: Unbalanced Consistency

- **Issue:** The dressing might be too thick or too thin.

- **Solution:** To thicken the dressing, you can add more mustard or a small amount of chia seeds, which will absorb some of the liquid and create a thicker texture.

To thin it out, add a touch of water or vinegar until you achieve the desired consistency.

Problem 5: Insufficient Seasoning

- **Issue:** The dressing might taste underseasoned.

- **Solution:** Taste the dressing and gradually add more salt, pepper, and any additional herbs or spices to enhance the overall flavor. Remember to adjust in small increments and taste as you go.

Plant-based Meals Planning Tips

1. Diverse Ingredients: Include a variety of fruits, vegetables, whole grains, legumes, nuts, and seeds to ensure a well-rounded nutrient intake.

2. Protein Sources: Incorporate plant-based protein sources like beans, lentils, tofu, tempeh, seitan, quinoa, and chickpeas into your meals.

3. Nutrient Balance: Aim for a balance of carbohydrates, proteins, and healthy fats in each meal to provide sustained energy and satiety.

4. Plan Ahead: Plan your meals for the week, making a shopping list to avoid impulse buying and wasting ingredients.

5. Batch Cooking: Prepare larger quantities of grains, beans, or roasted vegetables to use in multiple meals throughout the week.

6. Freeze for Later: Cook extra servings and freeze them for convenient meals on busy days.

7. Flavor Variety: Experiment with different herbs, spices, and sauces to add flavor and make plant-based meals exciting.

8. Incorporate Nuts and Seeds: Use nuts and seeds as toppings in salads, yogurt, or oatmeal to add crunch and nutritional value.

9. Explore Ethnic Cuisines: Many ethnic cuisines have delicious plant-based options, such as Indian, Mediterranean, Thai, and Mexican.

10. Include Leafy Greens: Incorporate dark leafy greens like kale, spinach, and Swiss chard for added vitamins and minerals.

11. Healthy Fats: Use sources like avocados, olive oil, and coconut in moderation to provide essential fatty acids.

12. Stay Hydrated: Drink plenty of water throughout the day and consider adding hydrating foods like cucumbers, watermelon, and oranges.

13. Homemade Snacks: Prepare your own plant-based snacks, such as trail mix, energy bars, or veggie sticks with hummus.

14. Read Labels: Be mindful of packaged plant-based foods, as they can still be high in sugar, sodium, or unhealthy fats.

15. <u>Mindful Eating:</u> Pay attention to portion sizes and eat slowly to recognize your body's fullness cues.

Everyone's nutritional needs are different, so it's a good idea to consult with a registered dietitian or nutritionist to ensure you're meeting your individual requirements while following a plant-based diet.

Balanced Plant-Based Meal

A balanced meal typically includes a source of protein, carbohydrates, healthy fats, and plenty of vegetables. Here's an example:

1. Protein: Lentils, chickpeas, tofu, tempeh, or quinoa.

2. Carbohydrates: Brown rice, whole wheat pasta, sweet potatoes, or quinoa.

3. Healthy Fats: Avocado slices, nuts (like almonds, walnuts), or seeds (like chia, flax).

4. Vegetables: A mix of colorful vegetables like broccoli, bell peppers, spinach, carrots, and tomatoes.

Incorporate a variety of foods to ensure you're getting a good range of nutrients. And don't forget to season with herbs, spices, and a healthy dressing or sauce for flavor!

Balanced Plant-Based Meal plan for Breakfast, Lunch, and Dinner

A balanced plant-based meal plan for breakfast, lunch, and dinner:

Breakfast:

- Oatmeal topped with mixed berries, sliced banana, and a sprinkle of chia seeds.

- A glass of fortified plant-based milk (such as almond, soy, or oat milk) for added nutrients.

Lunch:

- Quinoa and black bean salad with chopped vegetables (like bell peppers, cucumber, and tomatoes).

- A side of mixed greens with a light vinaigrette dressing.

- A small handful of nuts (such as almonds or walnuts) for healthy fats.

Dinner:

- Baked tofu or tempeh with a flavorful marinade or sauce.

- Steamed or roasted vegetables (broccoli, carrots, and zucchini) seasoned with herbs and spices.

- A serving of brown rice or whole wheat pasta for complex carbohydrates.

Drink plenty of water throughout the day and adjust portion sizes based on your individual needs and activity level. This meal plan provides a good mix of protein, fiber, healthy fats, and essential nutrients.

<u>Grocery Shopping for Minimalist Cooking</u>

Itemized grocery shopping list for minimalist plant-based cooking:

1. Proteins:

- Tofu or tempeh
- Lentils or beans (canned or dry)

2. Grains:

- Brown rice or quinoa
- Whole wheat pasta

3. Vegetables:

- Leafy greens (spinach, kale, arugula)
- Bell peppers
- Tomatoes
- Onions
- Garlic

4. Fruits:

- Avocado

- Lemons or limes

5. Herbs and Spices:

- Basil

- Oregano

- Thyme

- Paprika

- Cumin

- Salt and pepper

6. Condiments and Sauces:

- Olive oil

- Soy sauce or tamari

- Balsamic vinegar

- Nutritional yeast (for a cheesy flavor)

7. Nuts and Seeds:

- Almonds or cashews

8. Breads:

- Whole grain bread

9. Dairy Alternatives:

- Almond milk or oat milk

10. Snacks (optional):

- Hummus

- Rice cakes

This list provides the basics for minimalist plant-based cooking. Feel free to adjust based on your preferences and the specific recipes you plan to make.

Plant-Based Diet Meal Plan For a week

A sample weekly meal plan for a plant-based diet:

Day 1:

- **Breakfast:** Oatmeal topped with berries and almond butter.

- **Lunch:** Chickpea salad with mixed greens, cucumber, tomatoes, and a tahini dressing.

- **Dinner:** Lentil and vegetable stir-fry served over brown rice.

Day 2:

- **Breakfast:** Whole grain toast with avocado and sliced radishes.

- **Lunch:** Quinoa and black bean bowl with roasted sweet potatoes and salsa.

- **Dinner:** Grilled portobello mushrooms with quinoa pilaf and steamed broccoli.

Day 3:

- **Breakfast:** Smoothie with spinach, banana, mixed berries, chia seeds, and almond milk.

- **Lunch:** Hummus and vegetable wrap in a whole wheat tortilla.

- **Dinner:** Thai-inspired coconut curry with tofu, bell peppers, and snow peas served over jasmine rice.

Day 4:

- **Breakfast:** Vegan yogurt parfait with granola and sliced peaches.

- **Lunch:** Spinach and arugula salad with walnuts, dried cranberries, and balsamic vinaigrette.

- **Dinner:** Black bean and vegetable chili topped with diced avocado.

Day 5:

- **Breakfast:** Chia seed pudding with almond milk and sliced almonds.

- **Lunch:** Roasted vegetable and quinoa stuffed bell peppers.
- **Dinner:** Zucchini noodles with marinara sauce and lentil-based "meatballs."

Day 6:
- **Breakfast:** Whole grain pancakes topped with mixed fruit and a drizzle of maple syrup.
- **Lunch:** Lentil and vegetable soup with a side of whole grain bread.
- **Dinner:** Chickpea and vegetable curry served with brown rice.

Day 7:
- **Breakfast:** Breakfast burrito with scrambled tofu, sautéed vegetables, and salsa.
- **Lunch:** Mediterranean-inspired salad with hummus, olives, cucumbers, and tomatoes.
- **Dinner:** Baked sweet potatoes topped with black beans, corn, and a dairy-free yogurt-based sauce.

Another sample weekly meal plan for a plant-based diet:

Day 1:

- **Breakfast:** Oatmeal with almond milk, topped with berries and a sprinkle of chia seeds.
- **Lunch:** Chickpea salad with mixed greens, cucumber, tomatoes, red onion, and a tahini dressing.
- Snack: Carrot sticks with hummus.
- **Dinner:** Lentil and vegetable stir-fry with brown rice.

Day 2:

- **Breakfast:** Smoothie with spinach, banana, almond butter, and plant-based protein powder.
- **Lunch:** Quinoa and black bean stuffed bell peppers.
- Snack: Mixed nuts.
- **Dinner:** Zucchini noodles with marinara sauce and a side salad.

Day 3:

- **Breakfast:** Whole grain toast with avocado and sliced tomatoes.

- **Lunch:** Spinach and arugula salad with roasted sweet potatoes, walnuts, and a balsamic vinaigrette.

- Snack: Apple slices with nut butter.

- **Dinner:** Vegan chili with beans, corn, and bell peppers.

Day 4:

- **Breakfast:** Chia pudding with coconut milk, topped with mango and shredded coconut.

- **Lunch:** Hummus wrap with whole wheat tortilla, mixed greens, shredded carrots, and roasted red peppers.

- Snack: Rice cakes with almond butter.

- **Dinner:** Baked tofu with steamed broccoli and quinoa.

Day 5:

- **Breakfast:** Vegan yogurt parfait with granola and mixed berries.

- **Lunch:** Lentil soup with a side of whole grain bread.

- Snack: Edamame.

- **Dinner:** Portobello mushroom burgers with sweet potato fries.

Day 6:

- **Breakfast:** Acai bowl with granola, banana slices, and coconut flakes.

- **Lunch:** Mediterranean-style quinoa salad with olives, cucumbers, red onion, and a lemon-herb dressing.

- Snack: Trail mix.

- **Dinner:** Cauliflower and chickpea curry with brown rice.

Day 7:

- **Breakfast:** Vegan pancakes with maple syrup and sliced peaches.

- **Lunch:** Sushi rolls filled with avocado, cucumber, and bell pepper.
- Snack: Popcorn.
- **Dinner:** Stuffed acorn squash with wild rice, cranberries, and pecans.

Adjust portion sizes and ingredients to fit your individual nutritional needs and preferences. Always consult a healthcare professional before making significant changes to your diet.

Conclusion

Embracing a Healthier Lifestyle with Simple Ingredients

Embracing a healthier lifestyle through the incorporation of simple plant-based ingredients is a choice that not only benefits our own well-being but also contributes to the health of the planet. Plant-based diets are gaining popularity for their numerous advantages, both for personal health and environmental sustainability.

One of the key benefits of adopting a plant-based diet is its positive impact on cardiovascular health. Plant-based ingredients such as fruits, vegetables, whole grains, nuts, and seeds are rich in essential nutrients and antioxidants that help lower cholesterol levels, reduce blood pressure, and decrease the risk of heart disease. By focusing on these ingredients, individuals can actively improve their overall cardiovascular well-being.

Moreover, a plant-based diet can aid in weight management and even weight loss. Plant-based meals tend to be lower in calories and unhealthy fats, making it easier to maintain a healthy weight. The fiber content in these ingredients keeps you feeling full and satisfied, reducing the likelihood of overeating or indulging in unhealthy snacks.

Notably, transitioning to a plant-based diet can have positive effects on the environment as well. Animal agriculture is a significant contributor to greenhouse gas emissions, deforestation, and water pollution. By choosing plant-based ingredients, you're directly reducing your carbon footprint and contributing to the conservation of natural resources.

Creating meals centered around plant-based ingredients can be both enjoyable and creative. Experimenting with a variety of vegetables, legumes, and whole grains allows you to discover new flavors and textures. From hearty salads to flavorful stir-fries, the options are endless and adaptable to various culinary preferences.

In conclusion, embracing a healthier lifestyle with simple plant-based ingredients offers a holistic approach to well-being. By prioritizing these nutrient-rich foods, we can improve our cardiovascular health, manage our weight, and make a positive impact on the environment. Making gradual shifts toward plant-based eating is a step towards a brighter and more sustainable future for both ourselves and the planet.